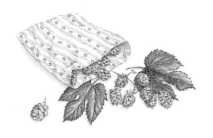

HEALTH AND HEALING
THE NATURAL WAY

THE STRESS
FACTOR

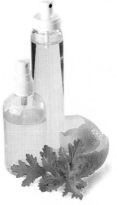

HEALTH AND HEALING
THE NATURAL WAY

THE STRESS
FACTOR

Reader's Digest

PUBLISHED BY

THE READER'S DIGEST ASSOCIATION, INC.

PLEASANTVILLE, NEW YORK / MONTREAL

A READER'S DIGEST BOOK
Produced by
Carroll & Brown Limited, London

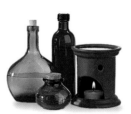

CARROLL & BROWN

Managing Editor Denis Kennedy
Art Director Chrissie Lloyd

Series Editor Arlene Sobel
Series Art Editor Johnny Pau

Assistant Editors Caroline Turner,
Madeleine Jennings

Art Editor Michelle Tiley

Photographers David Murray, Jules Selmes

Production Lorraine Baird, Wendy Rogers,
Amanda Mackie

Computer Management John Clifford

CONSULTANTS

Prof. Cary Cooper, B.Sc., M.B.A., Ph.D.,
M.Sc., C.Psychol., F.B.Ps.S., F.R.S.A.
*Manchester School of Management
University of Manchester
Institute of Science and Technology*

Dr. Adam Ward, M.Sc., M.B., B.S., M.R.C.G.P.,
M.F.Hom., Dip. Orth. Med.
The Royal London Homoeopathic Hospital NHS Trust

MEDICAL ILLUSTRATIONS CONSULTANTS

Dr. Francis Williams, M.B., B.C.h.i.r.,
M.R.C.P., D.T.M.&H.

Dr. Lesley Hickin, M.B., B.S., B.Sc.,
D.R.C.O.G., M.R.C.G.P.

CONTRIBUTORS

Susanna Dowie, Lic.Ac., M.T.Ac.S., R.W.T.A., Nancy Duin,

Siobhan McGee, Vera Peiffer, B.A.(Psych.), C.A.Hyp.

WRITERS

Richard Emerson, Sue George, Clare Hill,
Ursula Markham, Kate Swainson, Stephen Ulph

READER'S DIGEST

Series Editor Gayla Visalli
Project Editor Barbara Loos Chintz
Senior Associate Art Editor Nancy Mace

READER'S DIGEST GENERAL BOOKS

Editor in Chief, U.S. General Books David Palmer
Managing Editor Christopher Cavanaugh
Editorial Director, health & medicine Wayne Kalyn
Design Director, health & medicine Barbara Rietschel

Address any comments about *Eating for Good Health* to
Editor in Chief, U.S. General Books, 260 Madison Avenue,
New York, NY 10016

You can also visit us on the World Wide Web at
http://www.readersdigest.com

Library of Congress Cataloging in Publication Data

The stress factor.
    p. cm. — (Health and healing the natural way)
Includes index.
ISBN 0-89577-835-1
  1. Stress management. I. Reader's Digest Association.
II. Series.
RA785.S763 1995
155.9′042—dc20   95-20226

Printed in the United States of America
Second printing, November 1998

FOREWORD

Stress triggers reactions that are as familiar as they are unwelcome: a racing heart, sweaty palms, and feelings of panic. Although these involuntary responses are uncomfortable, they can save your life. If your heart did not pound and send blood racing through your muscles, you wouldn't have the energy to respond to certain stresses, say, jumping out of the way of a speeding truck.

In today's world, though, stress takes many forms, not just the threat of unexpected physical danger. Many of us face a variety of threats every day. These may range from meeting unreasonable deadlines at work, to coping with demanding children, to wrestling with financial concerns, to fighting traffic jams. The list is endless! While not life-threatening, these stressors can take a tremendous toll on your health, especially if they're repeated over and over. Research shows that unrelieved stress can lower resistance in the immune system, leaving us vulnerable to respiratory infections, back pain, hypertension, allergies, and a host of other ills.

What can you do about it? The answers are right here, in this book. In THE STRESS FACTOR, the causes of stress and its effects are examined and solutions are offered to the problems they raise. Understanding how stress affects your well-being is no simple matter. This is because stress is an individual phenomenon—what is stressful to you may be simply a challenge to your neighbor. To grasp the complex nature of stress, you must first examine how it manifests in your life.

In THE STRESS FACTOR you'll see how stress comes about in the family, the office, and the environment. You'll learn how to recognize the warning signs before it gets out of hand. THE STRESS FACTOR gives you stress-handling skills and demonstrates, in real-life cases, how others have successfully overcome stress-related difficulties. And you'll find easy-to-follow instructions for many natural therapies that will help you and your family keep stress at bay and ensure a healthier and happier way of living. Better living can be yours once you've mastered the secrets of coping with stress.

CONTENTS

INTRODUCTION: STRESS, A FACT OF
MODERN LIFE 8

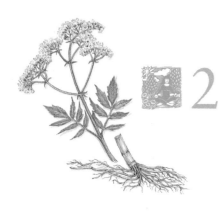

1 RECOGNIZING STRESS

THE STRESS RESPONSE *16*

STRESS: THE SIGNS AND SYMPTOMS *19*
The perfect mother 21
The acupuncturist 22

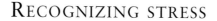

2 STRESS MANAGEMENT

PROTECTING YOUR BODY FROM STRESS *26*
A strong back 31
Alexander technique 32
Tai chi chuan 36

LEARN TO RELAX *38*
Muscle relaxation 39
Meditation 42

POSITIVE THINKING *44*

3 STRESS-RELATED DISEASES

STRESS AND HEALTH *46*
Working up to an illness 49
The homeopath 50
The chiropractor 52

ANXIETY AND DEPRESSION *54*
Yoga 56

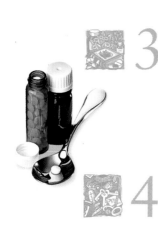

4 STRESS AND THE INDIVIDUAL

THE STAGES OF LIFE *60*

DAY-TO-DAY STRESS *64*
A woman of a certain age 66
Aromatherapy 68

TACKLING THE STRESS IN
YOUR LIFE *70*
Using assertion 74

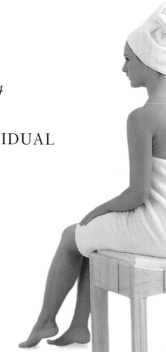

5 STRESS AND THE FAMILY

THE FAMILY UNIT *78*
A death in the family 82
THE COUPLE *84*
Sensuous massage 88
PARENTAL CONCERNS *90*
A single parent 92
A family divorce 96
Family therapist 98
THE CHILDREN *100*

6 A STRESS-FREE HOME

MAKING YOUR HOME A HAVEN *104*
Feng shui 106
Home health spa 108
HOME SAFETY *111*
CELEBRATIONS AND ENTERTAINING *114*

7 STRESS AT WORK

IS YOUR JOB MAKING YOU STRESSED? *118*
Body language 124
THE ENVIRONMENT AND THE
WORKPLACE *126*
Computer work 130
MANAGING THE JOB *132*
Public speaking 134
WORK UPHEAVALS *136*
An out-of-work executive 138

8 STRESS AND THE ENVIRONMENT

THE WIDER WORLD *142*
SAFETY OUTSIDE *146*
Visualization 147
MANAGING TRAUMA *148*
Post-traumatic stress victim 149
TAKING THE STRESS OUT OF
TRAVELING *150*
Overcoming fear of flying 155

INDEX *157*
ACKNOWLEDGMENTS *160*

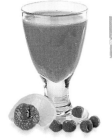

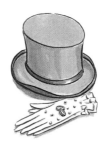

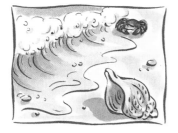

STRESS, A FACT OF MODERN LIFE

Potentially stress lurks in every corner of our daily lives. However, the challenges of life are not always a problem; it is how we react to them that counts.

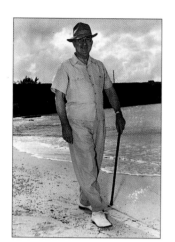

HARRY TRUMAN
U.S. President Harry Truman was known for his daily five-mile walk. It was his way to work off the pressures of the job. Walking is an ideal stress buster, which can be done anywhere, at any time.

LAZY DAYS OF SUMMER
Relaxing in the sun with a good book and a refreshing, cool drink is an ideal way to combat stress and relieve anxiety.

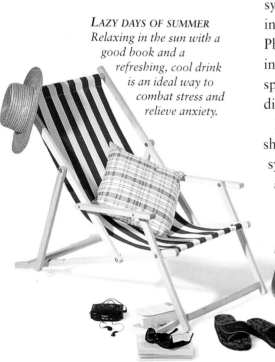

The traffic is moving at a snail's pace, and you are worried that you will be late to work. At home, the washing machine is broken, your inlaws are coming for a visit, and you haven't had time to start your Christmas shopping. Your neighbor's dog constantly barks at night, keeping you awake, but you do not want to risk a confrontation that might cause bad feelings. All of these situations, and thousands of others that are encountered in daily life, have the potential to generate stress. However, it is not necessarily the pressures of life that create stress, but rather how we react to them and cope.

Stress is difficult to define. For example, the stress of a crying baby will give some people a tension headache, whereas others will simply shrug their shoulders with a resigned smile. Our individual reactions to stress can be just as varied as what each of us perceives as being stressful. Some of the more common psychological symptoms of stress are resentment, anxiety, low self-esteem, inability to cope, lack of concentration, and feelings of isolation. Physical symptoms include loss of appetite (or overeating), indigestion, heartburn, sweaty palms, muscle cramps, and fainting spells. As uncomfortable as these symptoms are, they usually disappear once the stressful situation has passed.

However, this is not so if the stress is chronic. New research shows that continued exposure to stress can depress your immune system, lowering your resistance to illness and, in extreme cases, be a major factor in the development or aggravation of problems as wide ranging as depression, impotence, eczema, migraine, asthma, high blood pressure (hypertension), peptic ulcers, coronary heart disease, and cancer. An awareness of the ways in which stress can affect health is vital because taking too long to recognize the signs of stress may result in serious mental or physical harm.

WHAT IS STRESS?

Stress, as one writer put it, is "an associate of Strain and a consultant to Nag, having been referred by Job." Although stress is an innate part of the human condition, it wasn't defined until the 1930's when an endocrinologist named Hans Selye observed that his laboratory rats would develop peptic ulcers in response to various toxic substances. He borrowed the word *stress* from physics, where it means "external pressure exerted on a malleable object to produce distortion or strain." When people under pressure describe their feelings, the aptness of this definition is obvious—they feel pushed and pulled in all directions, crushed, wrung out, overloaded, at breaking point, about to snap. Their symptoms, however, often sound vague: "I'm not sleeping well"; "I can't concentrate"; "I feel run down"; "I can't cope with all my family's demands."

Stress is not a condition on its own, but rather a *reaction* to something, or what stress pioneer Selye called "an adaptive response to a noxious event." Selye invented the word *stressor* to describe such events. Typically, the most common causes of stress are unpredictable and uncontrollable stressors. But what is so fascinating and confusing about stress is that these uncontrollable events can be real (for example, a speeding car) or perceived (such as rumors of a job layoff). Either way our bodies do not recognize the difference between a real threat and a perceived one, and the stress reaction is the same.

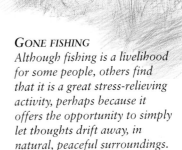

GONE FISHING
Although fishing is a livelihood for some people, others find that it is a great stress-relieving activity, perhaps because it offers the opportunity to simply let thoughts drift away, in natural, peaceful surroundings.

WHY DO WE EXPERIENCE STRESS?

Stress may seem a disease of modern times, caused by fast-moving, ever-changing lifestyles, but it has been with us since time immemorial. Our ability to cope with stress has been critical to our continued survival. In fact, our body has retained the same primitive responses that protected it from the kinds of physical dangers encountered during prehistoric times. Often termed the fight-or-flight response, this reaction prepared our forebears to deal effectively with threatening situations, such as a charging animal or a forest fire, by preparing the body to either confront the threat (fight) or to run from it (flight). To provide extra strength for a fight

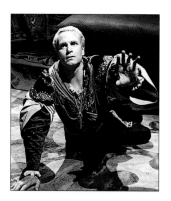

LAWRENCE OLIVIER
Performing or speaking in public is usually high on everyone's stress list. The actor Sir Lawrence Olivier suffered from such intense stage fright that for a time he considered abandoning his acting career.

SOOTHING MUSIC
Playing a musical instrument uses the creative part of your brain, diverting you from negative and stressful thoughts. It can also bring physical benefits, such as lowering blood pressure.

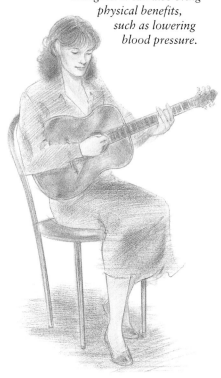

or the ability to run speedily away, various physiological changes occurred—a faster heartbeat, higher blood pressure, increased muscle tension, and quickened breathing.

Once we perceive the threat to have passed, our body relaxes—the muscles lose their tension, breathing slows down, and blood pressure drops to normal. Walter Hess, a Swiss physiologist who studied the action of relaxation on the body, considered the relaxation response "a protective mechanism against overstress." Indeed, that is exactly what relaxing is designed to do—help the body return to its normal state after the strain of either fighting or fleeing. In earlier times, the act of running from a charging animal would allow a hunter to expend the pent-up physical energy that a threatening situation evoked. After a stressful ordeal had passed, the physical response of relaxation is automatically guaranteed.

Men and women today face threatening situations that are usually of a very different nature than those experienced by our ancestors; however, our bodies have not updated our response mechanisms. We react to causes of mental stress—such as losing a job, the breakup of a relationship, or the unpredictability of public transportation—as if they were physical dangers. Our hearts race, our muscles tense, our blood pressure rises, to name just a few of the typical reactions to stress. In today's world, however, it is unacceptable to run away from a difficult meeting or vent your anger by slamming your fist into the wall. The result is an accumulation of stress that cannot be off-loaded by the physical activity of fight or flight.

GOOD STRESS VERSUS BAD STRESS

Stress is not necessarily all bad. It can occur in response to certain welcome events. Preparing for a vacation, going on a first date, and getting a promotion are only some of the many happy occasions with a large stress component. Stress can also be the vital spur that motivates us to learn, improve, and mature. We need a certain amount of stress to remain interested in life and to face challenges. Stress can even bring out the best in people, galvanizing an actor's stage performance or helping a student or worker maintain a keen level of concentration. Traffic analysts, for instance, take active steps to include stress-inducing elements in their designs of road markings at dangerous junctions to keep drivers alert. Without the spur of stress, people often succumb to boredom and listlessness.

While some kinds of stress are good, in that they improve concentration and motivation, others are harmful, inducing fear and anxiety that can be emotionally paralyzing. But what is the difference between good and bad stress? For one thing, good stress is accompanied by a feeling of being in control; bad stress arises from a sense of being overwhelmed by difficulties that you feel powerless to overcome. In short, stress is interpreted as good or bad depending on whether we feel we can control what is causing it and, if not, then at least respond to it with confidence.

REACTIONS TO STRESS

Thanks to research, we now know much more than we previously did about how stress occurs and why different people experience different levels of stress from the same causes. For example, those who experience a number of stress-inducing events—such as a death or divorce in the family, moving, or job loss or relocation during any one period—are much more likely to fall victim to illnesses than those whose lives over the same period have been relatively incident-free. Fortunately for most people, the stress accompanying such major life events, whether they are happy or sad ones, tend to be finite.

This is not the case with the less dramatic but constant, niggling irritations and worries that assail us, day in and day out. In fact, the cumulative stress of everyday concerns, what researchers refer to as chronic stress, can have as much impact on our health as stress produced by major life changes. Chronic stress can be caused by a number of things: worries about putting on weight, the cost of living, having too much to do, misplacing, breaking, or losing things, irritating noise, and constant interruptions. Luckily, while we may be powerless to avoid a major life-event, such as the death of a spouse or the loss of a job, we can modify or eliminate many of the little things that create chronic stress.

HANDLING STRESS

How stress affects you depends more on your temperament and your personality than on how many major life changes or minor irritations you are exposed to. Psychologist Suzanne Kobasa used the term hardiness to describe the capacity to respond positively to stress. There are three key elements to hardiness: *commitment*, or the strength of your belief in the value of who you are and the work

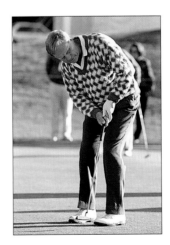

JACK NICKLAUS
Some athletes like golfer Jack Nicklaus use visualization techniques to help perfect their game and offset the stress of the crowds.

you do; *control*, or the conviction that you can influence the course of events affecting your life; and *receptivity to challenge*, or the belief that change and not stagnation presents opportunities for personal growth, rather than a threat to security. Her research showed that people with a high degree of hardiness were more resistant to illness than those who were less hardy.

In the early 1960's, two American cardiologists, Drs. Meyer Friedman and Ray Rosenman, discovered that personality played a huge role in stress management. They distinguished two broad categories of personality—Types A and B. Under this classification, people with a Type A personality were driven, competitive, impatient, aggressive, with a free-floating sense of hostility and a tendency to get angry easily. They also suffer from "hurry sickness"—a constant sense of urgency and a compulsion to achieve too much in too little time. Type B's lack these Type A traits; thus, they are more relaxed, more patient, less driven, they pace themselves and their work more sensibly, and feel less angry and hostile. While most of us are a mixture of Type A and Type B, those who are primarily Type A appear to run a much higher risk of succumbing to coronary heart disease than Type B's. Recent research, however, reveals that it's not the competitiveness or the hurried lifestyle of the Type A's that is harmful, but rather their free-floating hostility. One study conducted by Dr. John Barefoot of Duke University showed that doctors who scored high in hostility on personality tests were four to five times more likely to develop heart disease than low scorers.

Another important factor in determining how well an individual handles stress is whether there is adequate social support—that is, whether a person has both close and fulfilling relationships with a spouse, relatives, and friends. Researchers at three different hospitals in New York found that heart attack patients were at double the risk of suffering another attack in a six-month period if they lived alone rather than with a spouse or caregiver. The patterns of modern Western life often mean moving away from friends and family and a familiar community, and people who move away from their roots sometimes find it difficult to meet new people and make new friends. Research has shown that a lack of social contact and support can be a stress in and of itself as well as intensifying other stressors—circumstances or events that typically cause stress.

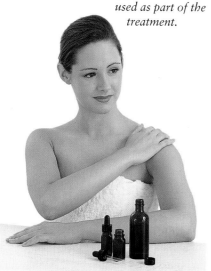

MASSAGING TENSION AWAY
Stress often manifests itself in muscle tension, and massage is a highly effective way to ease this tension away. Aromatherapy oils can be used as part of the treatment.

TREATING STRESS

Scientists and doctors agree that stress contributes to illness and that taking measures to reduce it will promote health. The problem for the sufferer from stress is how to choose between the extensive choice of countermeasures. The number and variety of the physical and mental manifestations of stress seem to be matched by the number and variety of ways in which people seek to treat it.

Modern Western medicine has little to offer when it comes to stress management. It is geared toward relief of symptoms. Often a doctor will prescribe tranquilizers or sleeping pills to patients under acute stress. Although they may help during a crisis or in the period immediately after a major stressful event, they do nothing to combat the problems of long-term stress. When the course of pills is stopped, or when the body builds up a resistance to them, the symptoms will return. Thus, an increasing number of people have turned to natural therapies—ones that address the causes of stress and the responses of the body as a whole, rather than using the stopgap measure of treating a particular symptom. In some cases people seek alternative therapies because they are wary of the possible side-effects of sedating medications and they do not want to become dependent upon them. Others believe that holistic therapies that emphasize the interrelation between the mind and the body are the most powerful antidotes to stress.

NATURAL THERAPIES

Strategies for beating stress using natural therapies are varied. Some practices are Western in origin, others Eastern; some are ancient, others modern. For practitioners of holistic therapies, balance and inner harmony are the key terms in the treatment of stress. These therapists seek to uncover why and how this balance is lost and help to restore it in the patient.

What the natural remedies all share in common is the desire to avoid treating specific symptoms and causes with modern Western pharmacology and medical practice, and instead to use techniques that take into consideration the whole person—mind, body, soul.

There is a multiplicity of stress therapies available with something to suit virtually everyone. Some approaches make use of herbal remedies, some involve manipulating the body to create beneficial effects, and still others encourage the adoption of corrective diets, exercise, and relaxation regimes.

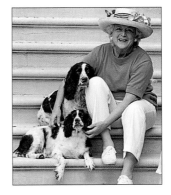

BARBARA BUSH
Former First Lady Barbara Bush is shown here with her beloved spaniels. Animals have a wonderful ability to help humans cope with stress. Studies show that the simple act of stroking a pet lowers blood pressure several points.

TONY BENNETT
One form of art may be used to replace another as a way of alleviating stress. Here Tony Bennett exchanges the stage for the easel, which is his way of relaxing from performing.

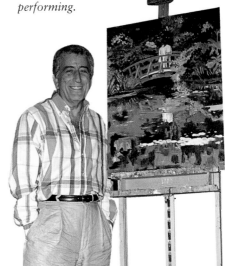

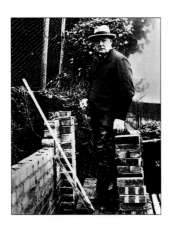

WINSTON CHURCHILL
Hobbies that engage both the mind and body are a wonderful way to offset stress. During and after the Second World War, Churchill devised an unusual way to relax from the pressures of public office. He took up bricklaying and built a long wall around the kitchen garden at his country home in Kent, England.

Our reaction to stress is complex, involving highly individual elements of personality, physiology, and psychology. The many ways in which stress shows itself justifies a very broad approach to its understanding, and a particular openness to the methods of its treatment. That the various treatments for stress pay a greater attention to the complete physical, biochemical, social, and emotional profile of the sufferer makes them at the very least a useful support for conventional medicine.

IN THIS BOOK

In *The Stress Factor* you will find a wealth of information on this fascinating subject. You will discover how stress affects your body and how it can impact, both positively and negatively, on your health, your marriage, your children, even your job. And you will learn a number of stress-relieving natural therapies that are sure to help you offset the impact of stress in your life.

Recognizing the signs of stress is not as easy as you might think. In Chapter 1, you will learn about the physical and emotional indications, and you can take a stress quiz to help you determine just how stressed you really are. Chapter 2 focuses on stress management and the ways in which diet and exercise as well as alternative therapies such as tai chi and meditation can help you deal with stress. Chapter 3 explores the link between stress and illness and looks at a range of natural therapies that can help reduce stress. Chapter 4 considers the role of stress at each stage of life and teaches you how to take control over difficult situations.

Chapters 5 to 8 provide a detailed analysis of how stress can affect four key areas of your life: family, home, work, and the environment. Chapter 5 explains how certain stressors can upset the family unit. Chapter 6 shows you how to turn your home into a stress-free haven. Chapter 7 explores the leading adult health problem: job stress. And Chapter 8 describes how you can guard against the stresses caused by environmental factors.

The Stress Factor contains a number of special features, such as case studies of how people have coped under various stressful situations. There are also descriptions of alternative therapies such as massage, homeopathy, yoga, and much more. The goal of this book is simple—to provide you with useful tools to help you combat the stress in your life.

CHAPTER 1

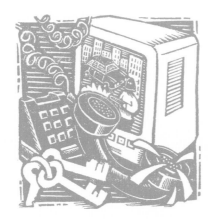

RECOGNIZING STRESS

*Some stress is a necessary part of life,
but too much can result in a wide range of
ailments and disorders. Fortunately, there are early
warning signs that can tell you when something is
wrong. This chapter shows you how to recognize the
physical, mental, and emotional symptoms of
too much stress, so that you can take action
before it leads to a serious illness.*

THE STRESS RESPONSE

The interplay between the senses, the brain, and the central nervous system allows us to respond instantly to danger, and once the threat to our safety has passed, to relax.

Stress is subjective, that is, different people will react differently to a stressful experience. How you personally feel depends on several factors: personality, hormones, or even the kind of day that you are having. Sometimes the same situation can cause feelings of stress one day but not the next. For example, if you have a plane to catch, and your schedule is tight, you may be fuming as you wait in traffic, worrying that you will be late. If your schedule is open and you can take a later plane, you are likely to feel much more relaxed.

Although the events that cause stress are subjective, what happens inside your body when you are under stress follows a set pattern, which can be objectively measured. Dubbed the fight-or-flight response, this reaction was first studied in the early 1900's by the American physiologist, Walter B. Cannon, at Harvard Medical School. Cannon discovered that when we are threatened, our bodies secrete catecholamines or "stress hormones." Produced by the adrenal glands, these hormones are known as epinephrine, or adrenaline, and norepinephrine, or noradrenaline. Their job is to orchestrate the body's reaction to stress.

FIGHT OR FLIGHT

When the brain registers a threat and catecholamines are released, they instruct certain body systems to shut down temporarily so that more of the body's efforts can deal with the threatening situation, either by staying and fighting or by running away. Also known as the automatic primary stress response, this instinctive physiological reaction gives the body extra power, speed, and energy in times of danger.

You are probably familiar with some of these responses to danger. For instance, if you step off the curb without looking and then see a car bearing down on you, your heart pounds and you breathe faster. As your heart rate and breathing rate increase, your blood pressure rises. Extra blood is channeled to the brain and muscles and away from the stomach and intestines— there is little point in wasting energy digesting a sandwich while staring death in the face. This shutdown of the digestive tract is experienced as a dry mouth because saliva production is decreased. To supply the extra energy you need, your liver releases energy-giving sugars. Blood sugar and cholesterol levels go up. Your vision improves. To cope with the possibility of injury, more clotting factors are produced in the bloodstream so that bleeding will be minimized.

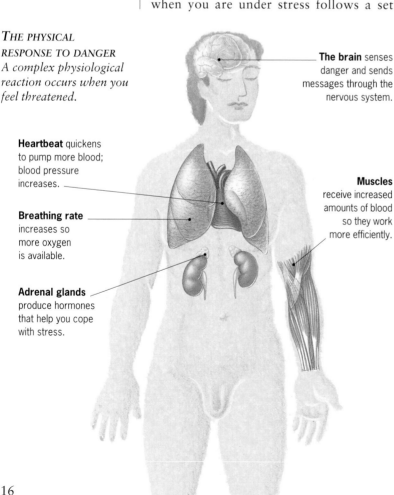

THE PHYSICAL RESPONSE TO DANGER
A complex physiological reaction occurs when you feel threatened.

The brain senses danger and sends messages through the nervous system.

Muscles receive increased amounts of blood so they work more efficiently.

Heartbeat quickens to pump more blood; blood pressure increases.

Breathing rate increases so more oxygen is available.

Adrenal glands produce hormones that help you cope with stress.

As a way of surviving physical danger—or helping others to survive—the fight-or-flight response is very effective. It can help people involved in serious accidents find incredible strength, if they need it to lift heavy loads in a search for survivors, for example, or to perform other "miracles" of effort.

GAINS AND LOSSES

The most efficacious aspect of the stress response, however, is also its main drawback—it is not under conscious control. The response is immediately set in motion whenever your brain perceives you are threatened. In an instant, this lifesaving reflex ensures that stress hormones are produced that put your body on red alert.

As an effective response to immediate danger, the fight-or-flight response cannot be beaten. But while the short-term benefits can be lifesaving, over a prolonged period this reaction can cause health problems.

In the 1930's, the Austrian-born endocrinologist, Hans Selye, was intrigued to find that his laboratory animals developed ulcers and weakened immune systems when they were subjected to noxious substances. What his lab animals were suffering from he called "stress," which he defined as a "non-specific response of an organism to any demand for change."

But what if the demand for change were continuous? How would an organism cope? To answer this question, Selye began to investigate the physiological reactions to such continuous noxious events as loud noises, bright lights, or extreme heat or cold. From his research he developed what he termed the General Adaptation Syndrome. According to Selye, there are three stages of reaction to continued stress. The first is the alarm response, marked by the stimulation of the sympathetic nervous system—heart rate speeds up and blood pressure rises. If the stress continues, the organism goes into the second stage, termed resistance, where the adaptive defenses are maintained but immunity is compromised. The final stage is exhaustion.

After analyzing the physiology of stress, Selye discovered another of its remarkable features. The body is unable to distinguish between physical danger and psychological distress. The worries, fears, and anxieties that are a part of everyday life can trigger the same physiological response as a brush with danger. If you miss the only train that will get you to an important meeting on time, your body will respond just as if the train nearly ran you over. In both cases, you will experience such physical symptoms as a racing heart, shaking hands, and dry mouth.

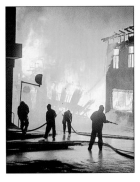

TRAINED FOR DANGER
Studies have shown that life-threatening jobs such as firefighting, can, in some circumstances, cause less stress than more mundane jobs for which people have not been properly trained or over which they have little control.

THE BIOCHEMISTRY OF STRESS

When your body registers that you are stressed, the frontal lobes of your brain alert the hypothalamus, a tiny section of the brain responsible for many bodily functions such as temperature, sleep, and appetite. During a period of stress, the hypothalamus engages in a feedback loop with the pituitary gland. The hypothalamus secretes a hormone called corticotrophin-releasing factor, or CRF, which travels to the nearby pituitary gland and signals it to produce adrenocorticotropic hormone, or ACTH. Once ACTH is produced, the pituitary gland releases it into the bloodstream, where it then triggers the release of the hormones adrenaline and noradrenaline (see page 16). These hormones are synthesized in the adrenal medulla—the inner core of the adrenal glands, which sit atop the kidneys.

This incredible relay system of hormones is responsible for setting off the body's numerous reactions to stress, such as rapid heart and breathing rate, dilation of the pupils, increased perspiration, and reduction of inflammation.

THE BODY'S RESPONSE TO STRESS
When stress occurs, the hypothalamus triggers a chain reaction of chemical and nervous system activities.

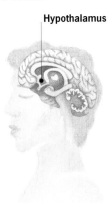

Hypothalamus

Hypothalamus

Pituitary gland

The best medicine

Two of the greatest natural ways to relieve tension, laughing and crying, may also work to keep the side-effects of the fight-or-flight response from harming you. Laughter helps soothe the body's nervous system and enhance circulation. It may also trigger the release of endorphins, natural compounds that mimic the action of morphine, which improve mood and reduce pain. Studies have shown that people who cry after major traumas such as a bereavement are more likely to remain healthy than those who refuse to exhibit any emotion.

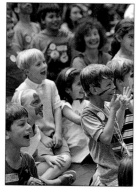

LAUGH AND THE WORLD LAUGHS WITH YOU The relief that comes from laughter helps the nervous and circulatory systems recover from stress.

If you were to escape by running from the train, your body's stress reaction would have been put to good use. And when the crisis was over, your body would return to normal. But when you miss a train and anxiety sets in because you will now be late for an important meeting, the body experiences no physical release, nor does the brain signal the all-clear. If this happens too often, over a long time, these stress reactions can cause physical damage and mental strain.

THE PHYSICAL DAMAGE OF STRESS

Researchers have found that the immune system does not adapt well to chronic stress. To function under the strain of chronic stress it simply works at a lower level, making people more prone to infectious diseases. In one landmark study, caretakers of loved ones with Alzheimer's disease were tested over a five-

---

THE EFFECTS OF STRESS ON PERFORMANCE

When people live with a constant sense of pressure, they feel on edge and stretched, and eventually become ill. It is well known, however, that some stress is necessary for optimum performance, and human beings need a balance where they feel energetic by day and tired at night. Although the right relationship between stress and performance varies with each person, the general pattern follows the curve shown below.

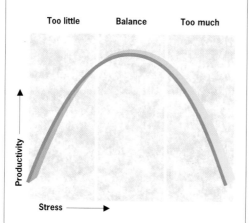

HUMAN EFFICIENCY CURVE The right level of pressure will spur you to work efficiently and productively. But pushed too far, you will make mistakes and your efforts will be counterproductive.

DID YOU KNOW?

In laboratory tests, animals exposed to high levels of stress produce endorphins, also known as opioid peptides. Endorphins are natural opiates produced by the body when under stress, such as childbirth or marathon races, to relieve pain and anxiety and induce a sense of euphoria. Some researchers believe that endorphins are so powerful that people can unconsciously become addicted to activities, such as long-distance running, that trigger them.

year period to see how this long-term stress affected their immunity. Compared to non-caretakers of the same age and gender, the Alzheimer caretakers came down with more colds and respiratory tract infections.

Because the fight-or-flight response unleashes adrenaline and other stress hormones into the bloodstream, where they surge through the body like a tidal wave, a number of organs are affected, none more so than the heart. Sudden, acute stress, for instance, can trigger such a precipitous rise in adrenaline that it can induce a dangerous and lethal disturbance in the heart's rhythm. The chronic activation of stress hormones can also lead to elevated blood pressure. Moreover, it is thought that a chronic oversupply of stress hormones can accelerate the build up of fatty plaque in blood vessels, including the coronary arteries and lead to heart attacks.

COPING WITH TENSE SITUATIONS

There are some individuals who seem better able to handle the physical challenge of stress than others. Athletes and people who are physically fit, for example, have lower pulse rates when they are under stress than unfit people. In one study, the pulse rates of a group of university students taking a major exam were measured. Although the pulse rates of all the students went up, the rates of the fitter pupils were slower than those of the others and returned to normal more quickly. It has also been found that people who exercise regularly run less risk of a heart attack. A number of researchers believe that the lower risk for such people occurs because their fitness is in some way offsetting any damage caused by the fight-or-flight response.

STRESS: THE SIGNS AND SYMPTOMS

Knowing the danger signs of too much stress can help you defuse its effects before your physical and emotional health are adversely impacted.

Since the early 1930's when Hans Selye developed the concept of stress, researchers have been trying to quantify and qualify the elusive nature of everyday stress. The first problem they faced was determining whether the stress was due to an external event, such as a missed bus connection, or because of some internal disposition, for example, a shy person having to go to a party alone. Stress caused from external events was somewhat easier to quantify. Researchers called these "life events." Two researchers, Dr. Thomas Holmes and Dr. Richard Rahe, devised a scale to illustrate the impact that life events can have on our health. Called the Social Readjustment Rating Scale, it ranked a number of stressful events. The death of a spouse, for instance, was rated 100; a major illness 53. Note that these events are seen as simply happening to people and are not the consequences of their personality or behavior. (For more information on measuring your reaction to life events, see pages 64–65.)

During such life changes most of us are aware that we are under stress and try to make a special effort to take care of ourselves by eating right and getting enough rest. But what about ordinary, everyday events? Why do some people get stressed out by little things, such as traffic jams, and others do not? Here researchers look at stress in tandem with a person's personality and psychological traits. Needless to say, this type of stress is harder to study because it is relative to each individual. For instance, an impatient person is going to be more upset about standing in line at the grocery store than a patient person. This type of stress can only be rated individually on a personal distress scale. Because everyday stress is so pervasive, finding out what rankles an individual can be difficult. To recognize the first signs of stress, look for nervous habits and mannerisms. Fiddling with one's hair or clothes, biting fingernails, foot tapping, and restlessness are all signs of stress.

COPING STRATEGIES

Stress can also be the culprit behind a variety of physical complaints. Notice that the symptom list in the column at the right applies to both acute and chronic stress. It all depends on one's temperament and personality. For this reason, researchers realized that they had to look at how people perceived the stress in their lives as well as how well they coped with it. What they learned was that stressors requiring active, conscious coping, for example, confronting one's boss or asking for help, were more likely to adversely affect a person's health than stressors that could be coped with passively, such as ignoring the noise from rush hour traffic.

Stress that calls for passive coping is not innocuous, however. Although we may not be aware we are under stress, our body is. One clue that we are passively coping with

DID YOU KNOW?
Up to 75 symptoms of stress have been recognized by Arthur Rowshan, author of *Stress: An Owner's Manual*. The symptoms fall into five different categories—physical, emotional, mental, spiritual, and social—and are often elaborately interlinked. For instance, arguing with someone can bring on a headache. This may keep you from sleeping, which in turn will make you irritable.

THE PHYSICAL SIGNS OF STRESS

A variety of problems may become manifest—all with their roots in the fight-or-flight response. The major areas affected are the muscles, circulation, and digestive system.

► *Headaches*
► *Teeth grinding, aching jaw*
► *Muscle spasms*
► *Aching neck, shoulders, and back*
► *Indigestion*
► *Nausea*
► *Ulcers*
► *Diarrhea or constipation*
► *Shortness of breath*
► *Heart palpitations*
► *Cold hands and feet*
► *Skin problems (acne, eczema, psoriasis)*

EFFECT OF STRESS ON BEHAVIOR

When people are under pressure, they may exhibit or suffer from the following habits:

▶ *Pacing and fidgeting*

▶ *Nervous tics such as wringing hands*

▶ *Talking too fast and rushing everywhere*

▶ *Hyperventilation*

▶ *Inability to relax*

▶ *Crying*

▶ *Constant fatigue*

▶ *Increased substance abuse*

▶ *Indecisiveness*

▶ *Insomnia and sleeping problems*

▶ *Increased eating and weight gain*

▶ *Decreased eating and weight loss*

▶ *Loss of effectiveness at work*

▶ *Recklessness*

▶ *Over-spending*

▶ *Increased smoking and drinking*

stress is a flare-up of a particular body system or target organ that habitually breaks down when we are under too much stress. For example, some people always get fever blisters when they are under stress, others develop headaches. Often a person's vulnerable stress spot is determined by heredity, for instance, psoriasis or hives. Lifestyle also plays an important role—old sport injuries often flare up during physical stress, such as a competitive game of tennis.

Try to become aware of how your body feels under such stress. Do you feel tension in your lower back? Are you not sleeping well? Is your stomach in knots? Are vulnerable areas acting up? For those who are under chronic stress, focusing on the physical symptoms is often the best way to recognize those events that are stressful.

INAPPROPRIATE RESPONSES TO STRESS

Another way to gauge how much stress you are under is to look at any inappropriate, self-defeating reactions you may have to it.

Comfort eating is one popular solution. Many people pamper themselves with sugary snacks when life is getting them down. While candy bars and the like will raise your blood sugar level quickly and give you a burst of extra energy and a feeling of satisfaction, this is quickly followed by an energy low, which can make you feel tired and irritable.

Smoking cigarettes is a common method of relieving stress, because it can make a person feel more alert and less anxious. But while the habit of smoking may be reassuring, it is so harmful that it cannot be recommended as a form of stress reduction.

Many people look forward to a drink at the end of the day. When used in moderation alcohol can make you feel less tense and more cheerful. A glass or two of beer or wine is relaxing. Heavy drinking, on the other hand, often leads to anxiety and depression. Additionally, heavy drinkers report that they are often unable to sleep or do not sleep well. With alcohol, therefore, it seems that less is more effective.

MONITORING STRESS

Because prevention is the best cure, it's best to be aware of personal stress levels before they become too high. The Stress Test on page 24 can help you assess the previous month's status. Keeping a daily diary of stressful times may enable you to pinpoint those situations that you find most troubling. Once you have identified them, you can take steps to eliminate them from your life, perhaps by changing your situation or simply organizing your time better. Or you may at least defuse problems by learning to relax or using the techniques outlined in the following pages.

In your diary you should write down how well you are eating and sleeping, and if you are drinking more than usual. You can also use it to keep track of the emotional signs associated with stress such as tearfulness or loss of interest in sex. This kind of diary will enable you to monitor how stressed you feel. Since stress is so subjective—something that you find easy to bear might cause your mate or a colleague great anxiety—you know best how you feel.

COPING WITH ALCOHOLISM

Job stress has been identified as a main cause of excessive drinking in men, whereas women are more likely to drink when stress comes from problem relationships. Because excessive drinking can lead to alcoholism, it is vital to learn how to cope with stress. One of the best ways is to talk about problems with a sympathetic listener.

In fact, the support group Alcoholics Anonymous (AA) believes that only by sharing experiences at meetings can members overcome their drinking problems and learn to live with stress.

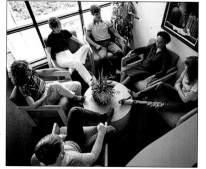

SELF-HELP MEETINGS
Founded in 1935 by Bill Wilson, an alcoholic Wall Street worker, AA is a well-known and respected organization that helps its two million members worldwide to achieve and maintain sobriety.

The Perfect Mother

Women who try to "have it all" are under particular stress. This may cause a variety of physical symptoms such as headaches and nausea that can be confused with a serious illness. As with all suspected illnesses, you should consult your doctor. Worrying about your health will only create more stress.

Penny has three bright children, a loving husband, and a job she enjoys. When her youngest child started school, she was given a promotion at work. Although her workload and responsibilities increased, she continued to help out with her children's activities at school, did all the housework, and cooked all the meals. In a few months, she began feeling tired and run-down, and then she developed headaches, neck pains, and nausea. She worried she was seriously ill and confessed her fears to her husband, Bill. He insisted she visit the family physician. After a thorough workup, her doctor could find no signs of any illness and said her symptoms were due to stress.

WHAT PENNY SHOULD DO

Her doctor explained that her headaches and neck pains came from her habit of keeping her jaw tightly clenched all the time, which is a very obvious sign of stress. He advised her to cut back on some of her activities and to take some time out for herself—and not feel guilty about it. It was vital to her health and well-being that she find other ways of meeting her responsibilities at home and at work without taking all the strain on herself. He suggested that she look for some ways of learning to relax, such as taking up yoga or meditation; he also urged her to ask her family for more help with the household chores so that the burden was spread more evenly.

Action Plan

WORK
Stop trying to pack every moment with activity. Learn to realistically schedule the day's activities—don't be afraid to let lesser things wait until tomorrow.

EMOTIONAL HEALTH
Join a hobby or support group, such as a Bible study group, a women's group, or a parenting group.

HEALTH
Learn some form of relaxation, maybe tai chi, meditation, or yoga. Take time out when stress is too much.

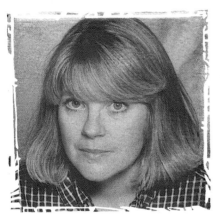

WORK
As responsibilities increase in certain spheres, the impact will be felt in other areas. Something has to give before you do.

EMOTIONAL HEALTH
Setting too high standards can make enjoying life impossible. It also isolates you from other people.

HEALTH
Your body is often the first to point out that you are taking too much on or are neglecting yourself.

HOW THINGS TURNED OUT FOR PENNY

Penny took a course in time management and learned how to prioritize her work and to delegate tasks to others. She analyzed her workload and asked her boss for an assistant, who has helped free up her schedule so that she no longer has to work overtime. At home, Penny assigned specific household chores to her children. Weekends became a time to relax. She started taking a weekly yoga class. After a few weeks, Penny's headaches and neck pain were gone.

The Acupuncturist

Many people visit an acupuncturist because of the stress caused by chronic pain. Using ancient Chinese diagnostic methods, the acupuncturist identifies the cause of the malaise and begins a course of treatment that can relieve painful symptoms.

PAINLESS NEEDLES
Many people worry that acupuncture will be painful, but because the needles are very fine and sharp, insertion is virtually painless.

MERIDIAN LINES
Two energy channels run down the center of the body, with the remainder duplicated on either side.

Gray:
Sexual organs

Black:
Lungs,
large
intestine

Red: Heart,
small intestine,
pericardium

Green: Liver,
gallbladder

Yellow: Spleen,
stomach

Acupuncture has been used in China for over 2,000 years, but was almost unknown in the West until the 1970's, when Westerners first saw photographs and films of people undergoing major surgery while they were still conscious. Acupuncture was the only pain relief the patients received, and yet they seemed to feel no pain. The secret lay in the use of very sharp, ultra-thin needles inserted at particular points in the body to redirect energy away from those areas of the body that were being operated on.

Intrigued by acupuncture's effectiveness as a form of pain relief, Western scientists tried to find out how it worked. They learned that according to the theory of Chinese medicine upon which acupuncture is based, energy moves through the body in set pathways, called meridians. During an illness, this energy, known by its Chinese name as *chi*, is not distributed properly. There might be a deficiency or a build up of energy, or the energy might be flowing too fast or too slowly. This theory made little sense to scientists at first, but as they investigated acupuncture, they found electromagnetic energy within the body that seemed to run along the pathways used by acupuncturists.

By inserting the needles into particular points along these pathways, the acupuncturist rebalances the flow of energy. Once the *chi* is flowing properly again, health is restored.

Origins

Acupuncture is said to have been discovered by a Chinese warrior who noticed a connection between the sharp arrow wounds he received during battle and the complete relief of pain due to several chronic ailments. Brought to the West by Chinese immigrants in the mid 1800's, it achieved little publicity outside Chinese communities until 1970, when an American journalist, James Reston, on a trip to China, experienced acupuncture-induced pain relief after emergency surgery. When he wrote about the experience in the US press, Americans took note. Since then acupuncture has

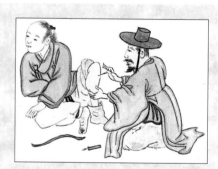

TREATMENT BY ACUPUNCTURE
Although it is Chinese in origin, acupuncture is also well known in Japan as evidenced by this picture.

been widely recognized, and even the World Health Organization has acknowledged its value.

Scientists still do not understand how, or even if, this rebalancing of energy works, and yet acupuncture is known to be effective in relieving chronic muscular pain and it may possibly help lower blood pressure and be used in the treatment of certain minor infectious diseases.

How does an acupuncturist diagnose stress?

Before treatment, an acupuncturist will conduct a physical examination during which you will be asked questions about your health and habits. He will also take your pulse at 12 different positions on your wrist, and look at your tongue. This examination will reveal your overall state of health and well-being.

How does acupuncture relieve stress?

Practitioners believe that a balanced flow of energy, or *chi*, within the body is the key to good health. They assume that when you are ill the body's energy is out of balance, and if they redirect the energy you will return to good health.

What stress-related complaints can acupuncture treat?

Acupuncture is particularly effective for stress-related illnesses such as sleep disturbances, headaches, and joint pain. It may also be used to aid in relaxation and depression.

What is acupuncture like?

Most people say that they feel little pain when the needles are inserted. The sensation is most like tingling. Sometimes, patients feel energy shooting from one end of their body to another when needles are inserted.

What will happen at an acupuncture appointment?

Once a diagnosis has been made, the acupuncturist will ask you to lie on a couch and to remove clothing covering the areas he or she intends to work on. During a typical session, an acupuncturist will insert one to 12 sterile needles and leave them in place for an average of 15 minutes.

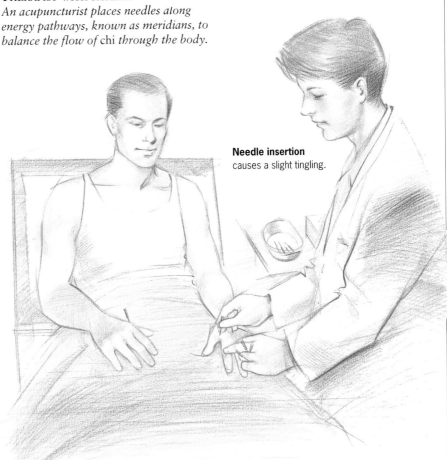

THERAPIST WITH PATIENT
An acupuncturist places needles along energy pathways, known as meridians, to balance the flow of chi *through the body.*

Needle insertion
causes a slight tingling.

One session may be sufficient but, typically, six weekly sessions are required before you see significant results. At the end of treatment, the acupuncturist may discuss how you can improve your diet or lifestyle.

How long does it take to work?

The length of time it takes depends on how severe the condition is, how old the person is, and how long the individual has been ill.

Are all acupuncturists licensed?

In 14 states, only physicians or osteopaths are allowed to perform acupuncture. Another 21 states require that acupuncturists be licensed, certified, or registered. For a list of practitioners in your area, you can call the National Certification Commission for Acupuncture and Oriental Medicine (NCCAOM) in Washing-ton, D.C. (202-232-1404).

WHAT YOU CAN DO AT HOME

Instead of needles, you can apply pressure to key meridian points to release blocked energy flow. Use your fingertips to press on the appropriate pressure point.

POTENT POINT FOR HEADACHES
Try relieving tension headaches by applying pressure to point BL 10 on the neck muscles at the base of the skull.

Press firmly but gently.

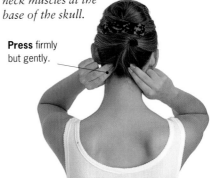

STRESS TEST

Listed below are some of the ways that people commonly react to stress in their lives. Think back over the past month, and on a photocopy of this page score each symptom according to your personal experience—3 if it occurred regularly; 2 sometimes; 1 rarely. Add your total and check your stress level below.

SYMPTOMS	REGULARLY	SOMETIMES	RARELY
Lying awake at night worrying about work or waking with disturbing dreams			
Overreacting to minor problems with anger, anxiety, or hurt feelings			
Overeating or a decline in appetite			
Increased use of alcohol or tobacco			
Long periods of boredom			
Unable to let go of tension easily; difficulty in relaxing, even in quiet moments, or finding that there is no time to relax			
Experiencing a change in sexual behavior			
Exhibiting a drop in performance at work			
Having difficulty setting priorities or making decisions			
An increase in the occurrence of any of the following: headaches, digestive problems, aching neck or back, breathing problems, heart palpitations, teeth grinding, muscle spasms, or a worsening of skin conditions such as acne, eczema, or psoriasis			
A greater susceptibility to colds or flu			
An unreasonably anxious need to improve performance at work, or unreasonable worry over seeking higher pay or promotion			
A frequent desire to consult outside professional help, be it from your physician, your priest or minister, or from counseling agencies			
Needing a great deal of personal support from friends and family, often more than they are willing or able to give			
Feeling rushed or that there is not enough time to get everything finished			
TOTAL			

RESULTS

15–25 UNSTRESSED

Suggests that there is not much stress in your life or, more likely, that you deal with it very effectively when it does occur. You should probably keep on doing what you're doing, as it works for you.

26–35 MILDLY STRESSED

Points to your experiencing high levels of stress at certain times, but that the feelings subside after a while. If you score 30 or more, you would probably benefit from embarking on a program for stress relief and relaxation.

36 OR MORE HIGHLY STRESSED

Indicates that your life has more than its fair share of stress, and that you are not coping with it very well. You should immediately reflect on your lifestyle and take action to make it more manageable and less stressful.

CHAPTER 2

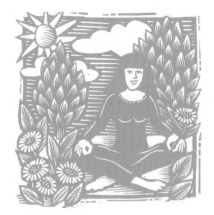

STRESS MANAGEMENT

In today's world, most people have to cope with the noise, pollution, traffic, and other hallmarks of progress. Luckily, minimizing the effects of these stressors on the body is not as difficult as you might think. This chapter reveals how an improved diet, an increase in fitness, and enhanced home surroundings can do wonders to minimize the damaging effects of too much stress. Better still, learning new and improved ways to relax will help keep stress to a minimum.

PROTECTING YOUR BODY FROM STRESS

You can strengthen your physical defenses against whatever life throws at you by eating and sleeping well, giving your body the attention it needs, and maintaining a tranquil mental outlook.

A body that is fit is able to cope better with stress. Proper nutrition arms the body with the resources it needs to fend off the increased demands that stress places on it. An inadequate diet, on the other hand, will deplete your nutritional reserves, leaving you vulnerable to disease. This in turn will cause greater stress because you won't feel that you have the strength to cope successfully.

Paradoxically, stress is frequently the culprit behind poor eating habits. In an effort to save time or energy, many people grab whatever is available, such as a hot dog, potato chips, and cookies. Typically, these fast foods are high in sugar, fat, and salt and low in nutritional value. Excessive amounts of sugar and fat can lead to obesity and put people at greater risk for heart disease, circulatory disorders, and diabetes. Too much salt can increase vulnerability to high blood pressure, which may already be a conseqeunce of high stress levels.

A HEALTHFUL DIET

Diet plays a critical role in helping the body deal with stress. In fact, stress quickly exhausts the body's supply of glucose, its major fuel. Once this happens, the body starts to break down the protein in muscles, a quicker source of energy than body fat. Therefore, extra carbohydrates are needed to provide fast energy. Fruits are especially good providers of quick energy. Next best are starches, or complex carbohydrates. Excellent sources are pasta, rice, bread, popcorn, and potatoes. Instead of giving you a quick surge of energy followed by an almost equally rapid drop, as do candy bars and other foods sweetened with refined sugar, complex carbohydrates are broken down more slowly into glucose. The glucose is then released gradually into your bloodstream to give you steady, sustained energy throughout the day.

In addition to extra carbohydrates, a greater than usual quantity of dietary protein, preferably from lean meat, fish, low-fat dairy products, and egg whites, is needed to prevent muscle wasting.

During stressful times the body has an increased need for vitamins A and C and for thiamine, riboflavin, and other B vitamins. Good sources are orange and yellow fruits

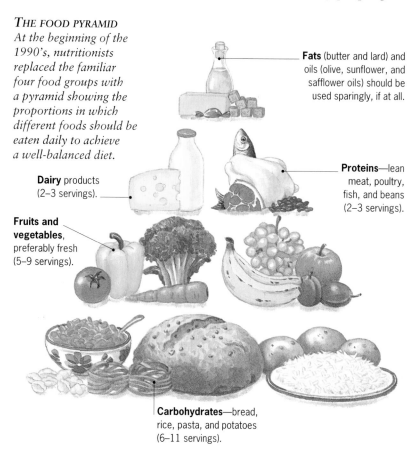

THE FOOD PYRAMID
At the beginning of the 1990's, nutritionists replaced the familiar four food groups with a pyramid showing the proportions in which different foods should be eaten daily to achieve a well-balanced diet.

Fats (butter and lard) and oils (olive, sunflower, and safflower oils) should be used sparingly, if at all.

Proteins—lean meat, poultry, fish, and beans (2–3 servings).

Dairy products (2–3 servings).

Fruits and vegetables, preferably fresh (5–9 servings).

Carbohydrates—bread, rice, pasta, and potatoes (6–11 servings).

DID YOU KNOW?

Because stress interferes with digestion, it's better to eat four to six small meals spaced throughout the day instead of the traditional three large ones. Also, certain foods that normally are well tolerated may trigger indigestion or heartburn. Fatty foods, which can be difficult to digest at any time, should be avoided. Many people also find that hot or spicy foods cause problems during times of stress.

and vegetables and leafy greens for vitamins A and C, whole-grains and milk products for B vitamins. Because stress also prompts the kidneys to secrete more calcium, magnesium, and zinc than usual, foods rich in these minerals should be increased as well. Select dairy products, tofu, oranges, dark green vegetables, and canned sardines with bones for calcium; nuts, bananas, apricots, and soybeans are high in magnesium; foods rich in zinc are shellfish, liver, wheat germ, and pumpkin seeds;.

Avoid or cut back on caffeine. While a little can lift your mood and boost energy, too much may cause palpitations and raise blood pressure (especially if you smoke), give you jittery nerves and insomnia, and trigger an anxiety attack. Coffee, tea, and many colas generally contain a significant amount of caffeine; to kick the habit, switch to fruit juice, decaffeinated beverages, and water.

In times of stress, it is more sensible to turn to comfort foods rather than indulge in comfort eating. Almost everyone has a favorite food, perhaps on that harks back to some happy time. For instance, homemade soup on a cold day may remind one person of being cared for in childhood. Another may crave a steaming bowl of oatmeal, scented with cinnamon and sweetened with raisins. Yet another may crave chocolate, which increases production of brain chemicals that have a calming effect. Experiment and go with whatever works best for you.

A GOOD NIGHT'S SLEEP

Sleep deprivation is one of the leading causes of stress; on the other hand, stress is one of the leading causes of insomnia. Extended periods of sleeplessness result in a lack of efficiency and make you tired, irritable, and short-tempered—symptoms that are only too readily compounded with stress. Effects of sleep deprivation were highlighted by a study of the sleep patterns of medical interns based in New York. Research showed that toward the end of the standard 36-hour work week, these young doctors suffered from short-term memory lapses, an inability to react to complex problems, and an increasing lack of concern about their patients. Research reveals that people who suffer from insomnia experience the same rapid brain wave patterns as people who are under stress. This may explain why falling asleep after a stressful day is difficult.

Getting to sleep

A regular routine will help you if you have trouble getting to sleep. Rising early in the morning, of course, will often make it easier to fall asleep at a decent hour at night. Part of getting a good night's sleep involves paying attention to eating habits, such as avoiding large meals late in the evening, as well as getting enough exercise. The more exercise you do, the more likely it is that you will sleep better at night. Start your exercise program slowly and build up the amount gradually. Be sure not to exercise just before going to bed.

A BED FIT TO SLEEP IN

Buying a good bed could be the best investment in your health you ever make. The place you rest your head must be conducive to sleep, not something that adds to your discomfort.

Buy the best mattress you can afford. A sagging, lumpy bed not only will be uncomfortable but also may lead to backache by not supporting your spine properly. Although the amount of give in a mattress is a matter of preference doctors say the firmer the better.

Choose natural fibers—such as cotton or linen—for your sheets and nightwear. They will allow your skin to breathe and will keep you cool in summer and warm in winter.

Use several layers of covers, such as a sheet and one or two thin blankets. You can always roll back a blanket if you are too warm; also, have one at hand should you wake up feeling cold.

STRESS-REDUCING FOODS

You may be able to reduce stress by changing your diet.
Foods and beverages you can try are:

▶ *Herbal teas, such as chamomile and peppermint, which have a calming effect.*

▶ *Foods high in vitamin B_6—yeast extracts, liver, whole grains, nuts, bananas—which have been claimed as stress preventers.*

▶ *Citrus fruits, bell peppers, and baked potatoes are rich in vitamin C, which helps your body maintain resistance to infection when under stress.*

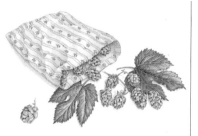

HOPS SLEEP PILLOW
To aid sleep, fill a pillow with hops (Humulus lupulus) or other soporific herbs carried by health food stores.

As bedtime approaches, do something that takes your mind off your problems but does not mentally or physically stimulate you, like listening to music, reading, or taking a warm bath. To ease insomnia, the old standby of a glass of milk and crackers at bedtime works. The reason is that a combination of carbohydrates (crackers, cereal, or bread) and milk increases the amount of tryptophan in the body. Tryptophan is an essential amino acid that synthesizes serotonin, the neurotransmitter associated with feelings of calm. A tryptophan-rich snack at bedtime can help induce sleep.

Other substances, however, may keep you awake. For example, the nicotine in cigarettes, which increases the secretion of adrenaline, is likely to make you too alert to sleep. The caffeine in tea and coffee is a stimulant; moreover, it can have a diuretic effect that may necessitate getting up to urinate at night, which will disturb your sleep.

Although many people believe that an alcoholic drink will help them sleep, this should also be avoided because alcohol disturbs sleep patterns. Like other sedating drugs that affect the central nervous system, alcohol slows EEG activity and depresses rapid eye movement (REM) sleep, thus inhibiting dreaming.

Remedies for insomnia

When sleep is not quick in coming, try pushing your worries to one side and visualizing a pleasant, nonstimulating scene, perhaps by doing one of the visualization exercises explained later in this chapter. If noise from traffic or aircraft—or from your partner's snoring—keeps you awake, try blocking it out with earplugs or consider buying an inexpensive white-noise or wave machine. These gadgets emit soothing tones to mask unsettling noises.

To calm yourself before going to bed, try an herbal preparation, ideally a tea. Herbalists often recommend particular mixtures, tailored to the individual, that can help you get to sleep. However, ready-made herbal teas can be found in most grocery stores. Chamomile tea is a well-known sleep inducer, so is tea made from the root of the valerian plant.

Should you still be unable to sleep, or if your mind is crowded with worries or depressing thoughts, see your physician, who may prescribe a sleeping drug or sedative. Such medications, however, will often produce an unsatisfactory, artificial sleep, and they can be addictive, which is the reason doctors usually recommend them as a short-term remedy only.

RELAXING FOOT MASSAGE

Built-up tension and a poor diet may sometimes cause painful cramps in your feet and legs, which can interfere with sleep. You can ease cramps by massaging the muscles. The massage will also gently stimulate the nerve endings on your skin, and your circulation will improve.

CAUTION
Do not massage your feet if you have a fever or any circulatory problems

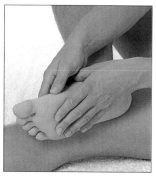

1 *STROKING THE FEET*
Place one hand on top of your foot and hold it firmly. With the other hand massage the sole of your foot, stroking with even pressure. Use smooth movements and cover the whole foot, from your toes to your ankle and then back again.

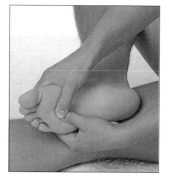

2 *THUMB PRESSURE*
Put one thumb on top of the other and draw them in a line down the center of your sole, pressing firmly. Then make similar lines on either side of the foot. With one thumb, press, using a circular motion, all over the ball and arch of your foot.

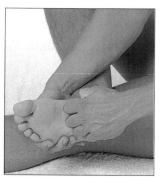

3 *KNEADING WITH KNUCKLES*
Make one hand into a loose fist; support your foot with the other hand. Ripple your fingers in small circular movements to make knuckling pressures all over the sole of your foot.

FINDING YOUR BALANCE

Getting enough sleep will not be sufficient to counteract stress if at the same time your body is full of the tension, aches, and pains from bad posture. Unfortunately, the human body is not designed to cope with an upright stance, and so can be easily damaged if held or moved in the wrong way, especially when standing. This is one reason back pain is the most common complaint that is seen by physicians.

Other parts of your body are also vulnerable. If you continually round your shoulders and back, you will squeeze your internal organs, making it harder for you to breathe properly and to digest your food. In addition, your hips, knees, ankles, and feet will have to take the strain of the weight imbalance to which they are subjected, and this can lead to osteoarthritis in later life. Exercising your back muscles will help you maintain your flexibility and ease the wear and tear on your joints.

Standing tall, looking good

An important aspect of good posture is balance. The slightest shift in your body weight produces reactions all over your body as it adjusts the center of gravity to keep you upright. Posture that puts you out

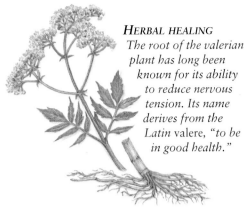

HERBAL HEALING
The root of the valerian plant has long been known for its ability to reduce nervous tension. Its name derives from the Latin valere, *"to be in good health."*

of balance can result in a painful lower back, aching feet, and a sore neck from holding your head at an awkward angle. All this is tiring and places a great strain on your body. Improving your posture will relieve this, and it will also make you feel more confident and alive. Good posture not only benefits your physical well-being, it can also do a lot for you psychologically. Standing and sitting straight and tall will make you feel more alert and active. This positive body language will communicate itself to other people.

Most human beings are born with good posture: just look at the way young children hold themselves when they sit on the floor. Nor is it something that people naturally lose as they age. Men of the Masai people in

Fashion victims

High heels tilt the legs forward and the body has to angle backward to compensate. When switching to flat shoes or walking barefoot after wearing high heels regularly, a woman may develop pains in her back and legs. This is because her muscles and ligaments have adjusted to the high heels and will not readjust readily to the lower heel height. You can compromise by wearing shoes with a 1-inch heel, rather than shoes that are completely flat.

A BODY ALIGNED

When people think of good posture, they often picture the rigid stance of soldiers. In fact, this chest-out-belly-in position may cause back pain by exaggerating the hollow in the small of the back, and putting too much strain on the muscles there. Correct standing places no extra strain on your back.

To stand correctly, imagine that there is a string running through your body and coming out the top of your head. Then think of someone pulling the string up and feel your body fall into line. Your hips should be held straight—do not tilt them backward.

If you find that when you stand, your weight is thrown forward, simply raise your toes off the ground. This will shift the weight back to center you.

To get your body into alignment, perform the following four steps.

1 *Stand up straight with your feet slightly apart. Sway gently forward until you feel your weight on your toes. Return to the starting position and sway slightly back so that the weight lies, correctly, in front of your ankles.*

2 *With your hands on your hips, gently move your pelvis forward. You should feel that this puts your body out of alignment. Now realign your pelvis, imagining your body weight passing through your knees.*

3 *Make sure your knees are not locked. If you can wiggle your kneecaps with your hands, your knees are relaxed.*

4 *Finish by stretching the neck gently upward, eyes facing forward, chin and jaw making a right angle to your neck, your arms hanging loosely by your sides.*

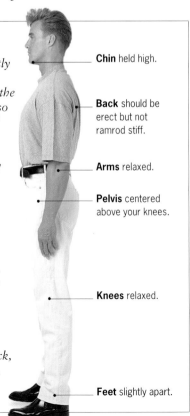

Chin held high.

Back should be erect but not ramrod stiff.

Arms relaxed.

Pelvis centered above your knees.

Knees relaxed.

Feet slightly apart.

SITTING CORRECTLY

Slouching in your chair can be just as damaging as failing to stand correctly. You should sit with your back as straight as possible, remembering the following rules.

▶ *Keep your shoulders in line with your hips.*

▶ *Keep both feet flat on the floor and balance your head comfortably on top of your spine.*

▶ *When reading, tilt any reading matter toward you so that you can sit straight.*

▶ *Position your chair and typewriter or computer so that you can sit straight, feet flat on the floor, with your forearms at right angles to your body.*

East Africa, for instance, can balance for long periods on just one leg, and women in some developing countries walk gracefully while carrying large burdens on their heads.

In the West, life is a lot easier physically, and bad postural habits are more likely to develop as people spend more of their time sitting—in cars, at desks, or in front of television sets.

Standing, sitting, and moving correctly are all essential parts of good posture. Therefore, it is an excellent idea to examine how you use your body from time to time. Think of how you sit when you answer the telephone, drive a car, read a book, or even just sit and relax. Do you hold your head on one side, pressing the telephone against your shoulder? Is your back rounded? When you sit at the dinner table, are you bent over? Do you twist your legs around each other? All these simple activities can strain your muscles, tendons, and bones.

Pay close attention to how you use your body at work. Incidences of repetitive stress injury (RSI) have skyrocketed because of the growing use of computers. Most repetitive stress injuries of the hand are due to the

carpal tunnel syndrome. Here, constant typing with the wrist in a cocked position causes numbness and weakness in the hands and fingers. This type of soft-tissue injury can be treated with anti-inflammatory drugs and rest. It is important to get prompt medical treatment for stress injuries, especially to hands and wrists; waiting too long will hinder recovery.

THE BENEFITS OF EXERCISE

Of all the natural stress beaters, regular exercise is one of the best. It helps dissipate tensions, makes you sleep better, and can aid concentration. Moderate exercise also has a beneficial effect on the heart and circulation, helping to ward off illness.

When stressful situations arise, you'll be better able to relax and take them in your stride if you are fit. If you quickly become exhausted in everyday situations, you will almost certainly benefit from exercise. Then, when you face additional challenges, such as moving to a new home or starting your own business, you will have the energy to handle it better.

continued on page 34

LIFTING AND CARRYING

The bones and muscles of the legs are strong and can be used to protect the back. Therefore, when you lift a heavy object, take the weight with your legs instead of bending over—and never carry more than you can manage.

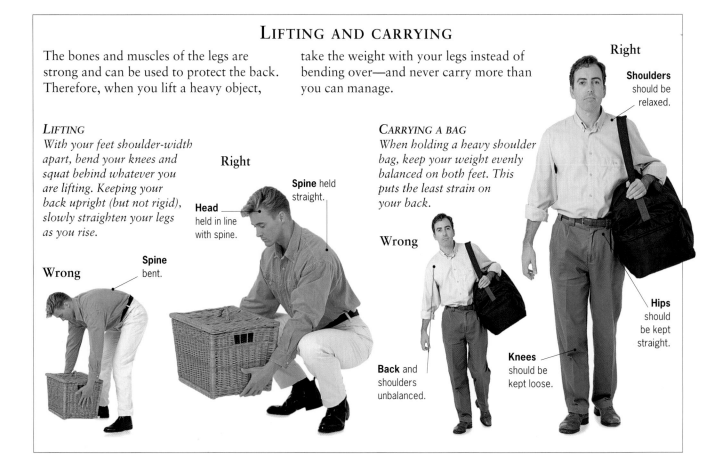

LIFTING
With your feet shoulder-width apart, bend your knees and squat behind whatever you are lifting. Keeping your back upright (but not rigid), slowly straighten your legs as you rise.

Wrong

Spine bent.

Right

Head held in line with spine.

Spine held straight.

CARRYING A BAG
When holding a heavy shoulder bag, keep your weight evenly balanced on both feet. This puts the least strain on your back.

Wrong

Back and shoulders unbalanced.

Right

Shoulders should be relaxed.

Hips should be kept straight.

Knees should be kept loose.

A Strong Back

Stress makes you mentally and physically tense.
This can quickly lead to back pain and thus more stress.
Appropriate exercises can relieve your aching back and
break the vicious circle.

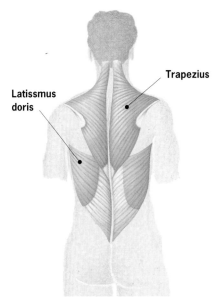

When people are stressed, they frequently feel as if the weight of the whole world is on their shoulders. In physical terms, this often means that people unconsciously hold the large muscles of their backs in a state of tension, and adopt a habitually slumped posture. Eventually they suffer from a painful neck and an aching back.

But back pain can usually be avoided by exercising to make your back stronger and more supple. A strong and properly aligned back will also improve your posture.

By becoming more aware of how you hold and move your back and then strengthening it and making it more flexible, you will ease any strain and free yourself from an added source of stress—back pain.

The exercises below are specially designed to help you keep your back functioning properly and prevent pain. Be sure to consult your physician before attempting them.

THE SPINE'S SUPPORT
Thick bands of muscle hold the spine in position, giving your body the flexibility it needs to twist and turn, as well as the strength to lift and carry.

SPINAL-STRENGTHENING EXERCISES

Start your day with 10 repetitions of the following exercises or include them in your regular exercise routine. Make sure all your movements are smooth and gentle to prevent jarring of your spine.

SPINAL CURL
Lie on your back. Bend your knees, then bring them and your head towards each other, tucking your chin into your chest.

Knees to forehead.

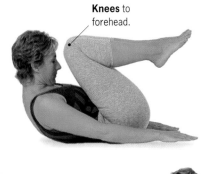

> ### WARNING
> *Stop immediately if these exercises cause back pain. If the pain continues, see a physician. If you have chronic back pain, exercise only if advised by your doctor*

SIDE STRETCH
Raise one arm, then bend to the side. Repeat with the other arm.

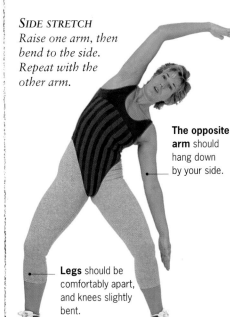

The opposite arm should hang down by your side.

Legs should be comfortably apart, and knees slightly bent.

SPINAL STRETCH
1 *Lie face down, with your arms at your sides. Raise shoulders and head off the floor. Hold for a count of five.*

2 *Cross your hands under your chin. Raise your head, shoulders, and legs, and hold for a count of five. You can also do this exercise with your arms stretched out in front of you.*

Head and neck should be kept in a straight line.

Arms should be by your sides, with palms up.

Feet should be slightly higher than your head.

Alexander Technique

Bad posture can become an ingrained habit and may lead to back pain. The Alexander Technique helps you avoid physical stress by teaching you how to use your body effectively, so that you can sit, stand, and move about in an easy, relaxed manner.

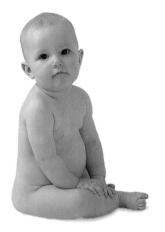

BACK TO INFANCY
The Alexander Technique helps adults recapture the free posture and graceful movements of childhood.

Babies have beautifully straight backs, but as people grow older, gravity and incorrect movement take their toll. Remaining in static positions for long periods—such as when sitting at a desk typing—makes back problems almost inevitable.

Over time, these poor body habits come to feel normal, but they place the body under considerable stress. Since the bad habits work against the way the body would move naturally, they are also very tiring.

The Alexander Technique aims to reeducate the body. In keeping with this idea of education, Alexander Technique practitioners are called "teachers" and their clients "pupils" or "students."

Origins

A professional orator, Frederick Matthias Alexander (1869–1955), found his career was in jeopardy when he started to lose his voice whenever he went on stage, only to regain it after the performance.

To find out why, he set up three mirrors, watched himself as he spoke his lines, and saw that when he did so he stiffened his neck, retracted his head, raised his chest, and hollowed his back. He found he could restore his voice by relaxing his neck, allowing his head to go forward and up and his back to lengthen and widen.

Over a period of 10 years, he gradually formalized his technique

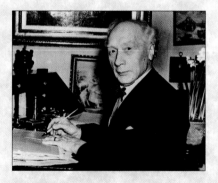

THE TEACHER OF MOVEMENT
F. M. Alexander traveled the world teaching his technique until his death at age 86.

of movement and posture, and taught it in Australia, the US, and the UK, attracting such pupils as the writer George Bernard Shaw.

What do Alexander teachers do?
Lessons are given on a one-to-one basis. During these sessions, teachers use their hands to align and direct their pupils' bodies, primarily concentrating on the relationship between the head, neck, and back. The pupil is taught the correct way to get in and out of a chair, to sit, to stand, and to move.

For instance, once you are standing as straight as you can, your teacher will correct your stance by altering the position of your head, neck, and back, or even changing the angle at which you may be leaning. At first, you might feel uncomfortable, but with practice, you should become accustomed to a new set of postures.

As your teacher realigns your body, she will repeat key phrases called directions, such as "Neck free, to allow the head forward, back to lengthen and widen." As you slowly relearn the correct positioning of your body, you will come to connect this with the directions, so that in daily life you can correct your own bad habits when necessary.

How many lessons will I need?
To see lasting results, a minimum of 20 to 30 lessons, each 30 to 45 minutes long, is recommended. Most teachers suggest three lessons a week for the first few weeks—after that, weekly lessons are sufficient. Some pupils continue to visit their Alexander Technique teachers for years to be sure of maintaining correct posture.

Can I teach myself the Alexander Technique?

No. You need the guidance of a trained teacher who can observe your posture and movements, assess any individual problems, and show you how to overcome them.

Is the Alexander Technique difficult to learn?

No, it just takes time to rediscover exactly how your body is meant to work. Some pupils find it difficult to avoid making unconscious muscular movements when their teachers guide their bodies into position.

How can the Alexander Technique relieve or prevent stress?

It reduces muscular tension and improves your breathing, thus helping you relax. If you can recognize when your body is not being used properly and when your muscles are tense, you can take steps to correct these faults. Teachers believe that virtually every movement you make can be influenced by using their technique, which can help you move correctly and stay comfortable while sitting, standing, or lying still.

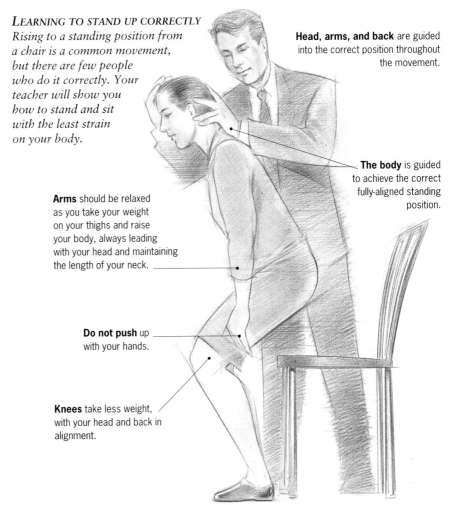

LEARNING TO STAND UP CORRECTLY
Rising to a standing position from a chair is a common movement, but there are few people who do it correctly. Your teacher will show you how to stand and sit with the least strain on your body.

Head, arms, and back are guided into the correct position throughout the movement.

The body is guided to achieve the correct fully-aligned standing position.

Arms should be relaxed as you take your weight on your thighs and raise your body, always leading with your head and maintaining the length of your neck.

Do not push up with your hands.

Knees take less weight, with your head and back in alignment.

WHAT YOU CAN DO AT HOME

To learn the Alexander Technique properly it is necessary to take lessons from a trained teacher, but certain positions can be tried out at home. Before you begin, make sure that you will have an uninterrupted half hour in a warm, draft-free room.

Wear loose, comfortable clothing, and as you practice, concentrate on the way your muscles and joints feel.

The semisupine pose is particularly relaxing and refreshing. When you lie in this position, your rib cage is relaxed and open, easing pressure on your lungs, freeing your breathing, and giving your internal organs room to relax. Also, your spine is well supported by the muscles in your back. This frees your whole body from the tension and muscular strain that are so often caused by poor posture.

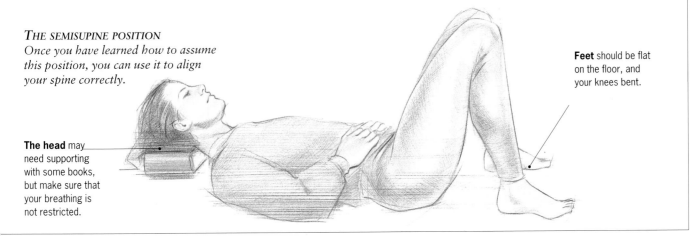

THE SEMISUPINE POSITION
Once you have learned how to assume this position, you can use it to align your spine correctly.

Feet should be flat on the floor, and your knees bent.

The head may need supporting with some books, but make sure that your breathing is not restricted.

Helping yourself

Exercise is one very effective way you can counteract the symptoms of stress. Among its other benefits, physical activity will burn up excess fatty acids and glucose released by the fight-or-flight response. Moreover, it will relieve muscle tension—for many, the hallmark of stress.

Various relaxation techniques (see pages 38–43) are also helpful for offsetting the effects of stress.

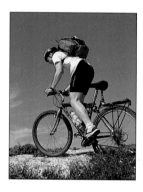

CYCLING TO HEALTH
A daily bicycle ride is a great way to stay fit, as it provides the benefits of aerobic exercise.

If you can stretch and bend your body easily, you will be much more resilient to the normal stresses and strains of daily life. To check how supple you are, try to touch your toes with your legs straight. If you can touch the floor in front of your toes, you are supple; if you can barely touch your toes, you could benefit from some stretching exercises; if you can only reach your ankles, you may want to start working soon on becoming more flexible.

Almost everyone can exercise, with very few exceptions. If you are suffering from a medical condition, are taking any form of medicine, or are recovering from an illness, always check with your physician before taking up an exercise regimen or a new sport. If you have been ill, choose a gentle exercise such as swimming with which to start, and don't push yourself.

Assessing your fitness

You can get a good indication of your general fitness by measuring your resting pulse rate; this is, your pulse rate when you first awake in the morning.

To take your pulse, place the tips of your forefinger and index finger on the inside of your wrist. Press gently until you can feel your pulse. Count the beats over 15 seconds, then multiply by four to get your pulse rate per minute. If your resting pulse rate is under 70, you are physically fit—the average rate is about 80. If your resting pulse is between 80 and 100, you are probably out of shape. You should see your doctor if it is more than 100, as you may have a medical problem. As your fitness improves through regular exercise, your resting pulse rate will fall.

You can also monitor your fitness by timing how long it takes your pulse to return to its resting rate after exercise. The average is four to five minutes, and the fitter you get, the shorter that time will be.

EXERCISE ROUTINES

According to the American College of Sports Medicine, aerobic exercise is not the only way to keep healthy. Research shows that just 30 minutes every day of mild exercise, such as walking or climbing the stairs, will keep you fit. In fact, a study done in 1993 showed that walkers had fewer cold symptoms than nonwalkers. Although an increase in strength is important, improving

endurance will probably help you the most in coping with stress. Brisk walking and cycling, for instance, are excellent ways to improve stamina, so instead of going by car, plan to make your shopping trips and other journeys on foot or by bike. If you have far to go, park the car or leave the train or bus some distance from your destination and walk the rest of the way.

You can also increase your fitness as you perform chores around the house and in the yard. Gardening, especially heavy digging, will strengthen your arms and legs, while vacuuming and making beds contribute to flexibility and strength, but take care not to strain your back. Take good care of your back by practicing bending, lifting, and carrying correctly (see page 30).

Many sports and hobbies, such as swimming, dancing, and hiking, have physical benefits as well as being relaxing and stress reducing in themselves. Make exercise part of your social life—a weekly swim with a friend, for example.

Exercising regularly

For people who need the discipline of a formal exercise program or simply like the idea of exercising with others, most communities have recreation centers where exercise classes are held. Or you can carry out a simple but effective program in your own home.

It would be counterproductive, however, to take up any form of exercise that you do not enjoy. A boring routine will soon be dropped. To avoid boredom, combine activities—such as exercising in a class and

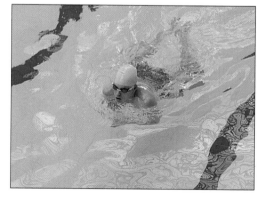

AN IDEAL EXERCISE ENVIRONMENT
Whether you swim or perform exercises in the shallow end of a pool, water offers resistance, thereby increasing the amount of energy you use up. It also reduces the gravitational pull on your body, taking the strain off muscles and joints.

swimming one or two evenings a week, or taking a brisk walk at lunchtime and bike riding on the weekend.

When you exercise is a matter of individual preference. Some people like to do it first thing in the morning, while others find evenings preferable, particularly if the day has been emotionally stressful. Working the frustration out at night can be a great release.

The rule for all exercise is never to attempt too much too quickly. Studies show that heart attacks occur more frequently during, or after, strenuous physical activity in a person who has been sedentary. This holds for the couch potato who suddenly decides to work out and overdoes it, or the

weekend athlete who has returned to sports after missing a few weeks. The reason that exercise can trigger a heart attack in the physically unfit is not clear; some researchers think that the sudden rise in heart rate and blood pressure disrupts plaque in the heart's arteries, causing a blockage.

When you begin to exercise, start slowly, especially if you have not worked out in a while. Begin by finding a level of exercise that is comfortable for you and stay at that level for at least a week. Then slowly increase the difficulty or length of time. Also, be sure to start off any activity with a gentle warm-up and allow five minutes of cooling-down exercises at the end.

EXERCISING SUCCESSFULLY

To get the most out of exercise, bear these points in mind.

▶ *Exercise should not hurt. If it does, stop.*

▶ *Fresh air is healthy, so exercise outdoors as much as possible.*

▶ *Replace liquid lost from your body during exercise by drinking plenty of water.*

A GENTLE EXERCISE ROUTINE

Aerobic exercise is any sustained movement that makes your heart beat faster and increases stamina by conditioning the heart, lungs, and muscles. It improves circulation so that more oxygen reaches the brain cells, and it may stimulate the production of endorphins, which are the body's own "feel good" chemicals. Do the following gentle routine for no more than 15 minutes,

with a 1-minute march between each stage. You can use the regimen to get off to a good start in the morning or to banish workday stress in the evening. Be sure to wear sports shoes and comfortable clothes.

These exercises can be adapted easily to your own level of fitness, but if you are over 40 and do not usually exercise, check with your physician before starting the program.

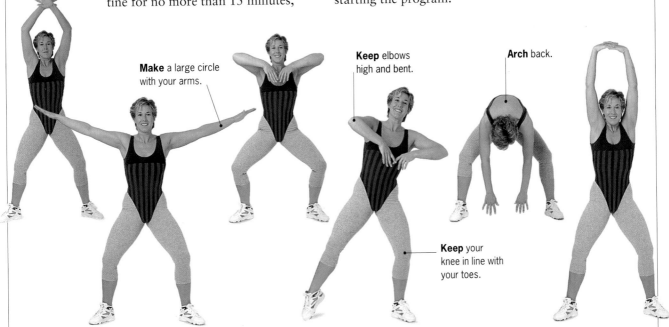

Make a large circle with your arms.

Keep elbows high and bent.

Arch back.

Keep your knee in line with your toes.

1 *With your feet apart and your knees bent, swing your arms up over your head, breathing in deeply. As you breathe out, bring your arms down slowly and cross them in front of you. Repeat exercise 3 times.*

2 *Stand with your feet apart and your knees bent. Bend your elbows up and push off to either side, moving your weight over alternate feet, coming back to the center each time. Meanwhile, move your elbows back and forward to stretch your chest muscles. Repeat exercise 20 times.*

3 *With your feet apart and your knees slightly bent, drop your torso forward. Interlock your fingers, then stretch your arms and body up, palms to the ceiling. Hold briefly, then drop your torso forward and swing gently. Now slowly stand, straightening your spine. Repeat exercise 3 times.*

Tai Chi Chuan

Tai chi chuan, also known as tai ji quan, is a combination of exercise, Chinese medicine, and Oriental philosophy. Called tai chi (or tai ji) for short, its slow, harmonious movements can help people relax and alleviate stress.

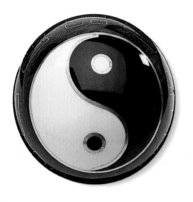

YIN AND YANG
According to the Chinese philosophy, Taoism, all things under the sun consist of a mixture of two principles: yin (the earth, passive, dark, and feminine) and yang (the heavens, active, bright, and masculine).

Watching a group of people slowly and gracefully going through the precise movements that comprise tai chi, you can hardly believe that this is one of the martial arts—but, when performed at lightning speed by an expert, it can inflict a great deal of damage. Today, however, tai chi is primarily practiced to reduce stress, increase overall tone and flexibility, and achieve inner harmony.

What does tai chi consist of?
There are a number of styles of tai chi. The most common one in the West has two forms: a short one of about 40 movements, which, when learned thoroughly, takes about 10 minutes to perform; and a long one with over 100 movements, which takes about 25 minutes. The movements are precise, and there are many rules on how to hold the body. You need to carry out each exercise very slowly—in fact the slower the better, as long as balance can be maintained. This will give you time to examine all parts of your body to ensure you are doing a particular movement correctly. Your teacher will instruct you in how to blend each movement into the next in a continuous flow.

How does tai chi reduce stress?
Tai chi is a form of meditation in motion. It calms the mind and helps disperse negative thoughts. The deep slow breathing that is practiced helps to induce a state of relaxation. As you concentrate on the feel of the balances and imbalances of your body while your body flows from one movement to another, you lose track of the outside world and its worries. In addition, tai chi demands natural movement, and muscle tension is released as you step forward and back, turn, swing around, and bend with coordinated arm movements.

Does tai chi improve fitness?
Adherents believe that the movements improve the flow of the body's natural energy, *chi*, along various meridians (see page 22). The movements exercise all the joints of the body, increasing flexibility. Because

Origins

Tai chi has its philosophical roots in Taoism, which can be traced back to China in the sixth century B.C. Taoism emphasizes patience, simplicity, and harmony with nature, and states that all things are composed of different combinations of the two complementary forces, yin and yang. Yin represents yielding and evasion; yang denotes firmness and resistance.

According to tradition, the Taoist philosopher, Chang Sen-feng, dreamed of a snake being stabbed by a crane. As the snake alternately evaded and resisted the crane's bill, Chang saw these animals as the embodiment of yin and yang, and from this he devised the first series of movements that eventually became

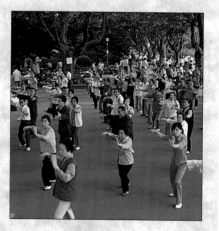

TAI CHI IN SHANGHAI
The relaxed and graceful tai chi exercises are often performed by groups outdoors in a park.

tai chi. In 1956, the Chinese government, under Chairman Mao, standardized tai chi into 24 movements.

it is performed in slow motion, tai chi calls for deep breathing, which increases the amount of oxygen going to the heart, and improves the capacity of the lungs.

Can anyone learn tai chi?
Tai chi is suitable for virtually everyone. Because it improves blood and lymph circulation, it is ideal for those in poor health. However, if you have back or joint problems, check with your doctor before starting.

Can I teach myself tai chi?
No. Tai chi teachers emphasize that the only way to learn properly is by watching a physical demonstration of the movements. Personal guidance is essential for learning correct body alignment and maintaining mental and physical concentration. But after lessons with an experienced teacher you can, and should, practice tai chi on your own.

Does it take long to learn tai chi?
If you take a weekly one-hour class, it will take 12 to 18 months to learn and remember all the 100 or so movements of the long form of tai chi. Attending more often will speed up this process, but it can take decades to become an expert.

What are the classes like?
Initially, you will be in a class of beginners, all learning the movements for the first time. Later, you may attend classes with students of different abilities. The teacher may have you carry out a sequence you have learned, then teach you the next few movements to work on for the rest of the class, or he will take the entire class back to an earlier sequence to perfect their style. If you want individual attention, it is best to join a class that has fewer than a dozen people.

WHAT YOU CAN DO AT HOME

These exercises are the beginning of a series of movements called "Heaven and earth". Wear loose clothing; go barefoot or wear socks or slippers.

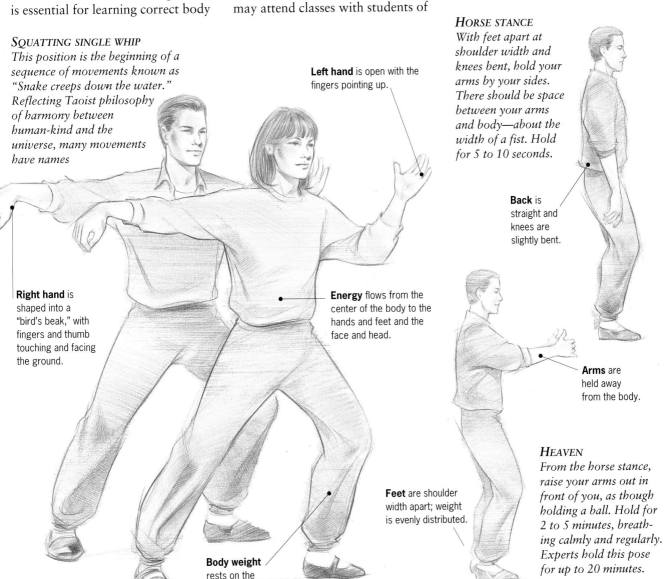

SQUATTING SINGLE WHIP
This position is the beginning of a sequence of movements known as "Snake creeps down the water." Reflecting Taoist philosophy of harmony between human-kind and the universe, many movements have names

Left hand is open with the fingers pointing up.

Right hand is shaped into a "bird's beak," with fingers and thumb touching and facing the ground.

Energy flows from the center of the body to the hands and feet and the face and head.

Body weight rests on the left leg.

Feet are shoulder width apart; weight is evenly distributed.

HORSE STANCE
With feet apart at shoulder width and knees bent, hold your arms by your sides. There should be space between your arms and body—about the width of a fist. Hold for 5 to 10 seconds.

Back is straight and knees are slightly bent.

Arms are held away from the body.

HEAVEN
From the horse stance, raise your arms out in front of you, as though holding a ball. Hold for 2 to 5 minutes, breathing calmly and regularly. Experts hold this pose for up to 20 minutes.

LEARN TO RELAX

When you are anxious, your body becomes tense. Relaxation techniques can help you feel calmer and more controlled. Use them at least once a day, to turn off the pressure.

Is television relaxing?
Many people list watching television as their favorite method of relaxation. But whether it really is depends very much on what they watch. Viewing a romantic film or a comedy can be both enjoyable and stress reducing. Studies have shown, however, that watching violent programs does little or nothing to lessen anxiety and stress; in fact, it can have the opposite effect. In addition, compared with people who use different forms of relaxation, television addicts are more likely to mistrust others and see the world as a hostile place.

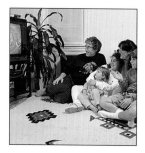

RELAXING AT HOME
A family may often feel that the only time they get to relax together is when they are watching television.

No matter what makes you feel stressed out—your boss in a bad mood, your children misbehaving, having to admit to making a mistake, or trying to deal with bumper-to-bumper traffic—you need to find a way of relieving the pressure.

One of the most effective ways of curbing stress is to relax. But purposeful relaxation is more than putting your feet up and watching television. It the conscious turning off of everyday worries. The results can be highly therapeutic and beneficial for both mind and body.

DIFFERENT WAYS OF RELAXING
Relaxation itself is as subjective an experience as stress. Just as there are stressors that evoke different reactions, there are ways to relax that, depending on your personal makeup, provide varying degrees of relaxation. Going for a walk, gardening, taking a bath, or enjoying a quiet evening at home with friends are well-known relaxing activities. You can add to the list reading, going out for dinner, writing to a friend, and watching a video of an old movie. At the very least, these reassuring activities will take your mind off your problems.

Although it does not really matter where you relax, safety, peace, and quiet are essential. You could, for example, watch the world go by in the local park during your lunch break or meditate in the evening at home. A change of scenery can be relaxing in itself. If you work indoors all day, go outside for a walk. If the walk is brisk, you will have an added aerobic benefit. This will help improve sleep patterns (see page 27) and increase your resistance to stress. If you work away from home, getting home and sitting down in your favorite chair with a book or newspaper can be relaxing. Gentle stretching exercises can also ease tension.

BIOFEEDBACK
For many people, the simple act of relaxation needs to be relearned. One excellent way is to use biofeedback to teach you how your body feels when it is stressed and how it feels when it is relaxed.

In this procedure, electrodes are placed on various parts of your body, for example, the scalp to measure muscle tension, or fingers, to measure body temperature; the electrodes are then connected to a piece of equipment (typically no bigger than a small radio) which is called the biofeedback monitor. The monitor registers changes in body functions, such as slight variations in heart rate, blood pressure, skin temperature, or minute amounts of perspiration on the skin. These

THE BODY RELAXING
As your body relaxes, changes take place that help to increase your physical and mental resistance to everyday pressure.

Brain wave patterns change.

Saliva production increases to aid digestion.

Skin temperature rises.

Heart rate and blood pressure drop.

Stomach— normal blood supply returns.

Muscle Relaxation

Learn to ease the tensions of daily life through deep breathing and progressive muscle relaxation. Easy to master and beneficial for all ages, this routine can help relieve your tensions and enhance your life.

Complete physical and mental relaxation can rarely be achieved simply by putting your feet up. When stress has been prolonged, or if there is a related condition such as high blood pressure, you may need to take positive steps toward reducing tension.

You can combine deep breathing with simple muscle-relaxing exercises to get the maximum benefit in the shortest possible time. It is best to practice this routine as frequently as possible. Regular relaxation has a cumulative effect, and the more you do it, the more quickly you will be able to enter a state of deep

relaxation, and the longer its effects will last. All that is needed is the discipline and dedication to integrate it into your life.

Ideally, you should perform progressive muscle relaxation exercises twice a day. Choose a time when you are feeling alert; do not do the exercises when you are tired, as you might become so relaxed that you fall asleep.

You should soon find that, after practicing these relaxation exercises, you feel a great deal more at ease and better able to deal with daily stresses and tensions.

DEEP BREATHING

When you're tense, your breathing becomes shallow. Therefore, a simple and effective method of reducing tension is to breathe deeply and regularly.

One method of deep breathing is called *pranayama*, which is a form of yoga. People who practice pranayama believe that by taking full, deep breaths, you absorb more life energy or *prana* from the atmosphere.

To practice deep breathing, place your hands flat on the area just above your navel. Inhale, raising your belly and pushing out your hands. Exhale, pulling in your belly beneath your hands. Repeat.

PROGRESSIVE MUSCLE RELAXATION

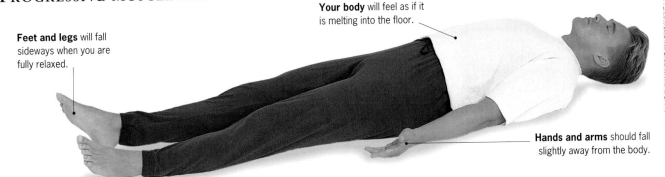

Your body will feel as if it is melting into the floor.

Feet and legs will fall sideways when you are fully relaxed.

Hands and arms should fall slightly away from the body.

Lie down in a warm room and close your eyes to help your concentration. Breathe in and out deeply for two or three minutes to establish a regular pattern of respiration. Follow the sequence (right), tensing each part of your body in turn without involving any other muscles.

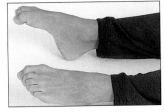

1 *Tense your feet and toes hard. Hold for a moment, then relax. Now tense your calf muscles; hold for a moment, then slowly relax.*

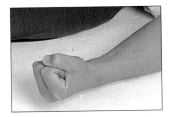

2 *Continue in the same way in the following order: thighs, abdomen, chest, hands, arms, shoulders, neck, jaw, and face.*

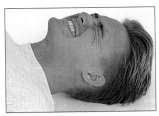

3 *Clench your teeth and shut your eyes tightly so that the muscles of your face are tense. Then relax them, and feel your face soften.*

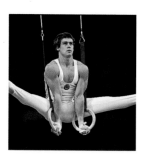

WINNING THOUGHTS
Many top athletes use positive visualization (see opposite page) to excel in their chosen fields. Imagining performing a routine perfectly may help ensure success.

changes are not consciously felt, as a rule, but when they are monitored by biofeedback machines, they can provide many meaningful clues to the ways in which your body registers stress.

Listening to your body

During a biofeedback session, meter readouts or tones will tell you whether the tension in your scalp muscles or your body temperature is increasing or decreasing. However, by visualizing a pleasant scene, concentrating on a piece of lyrical music, or repeating a mantra or affirmation, for example, or by using some other relaxation technique, you can reduce your stress level and muscle tension. This mental effort will reduce the number on the meter readout or lower the sound. Biofeedback only makes your stress visible or audible; it is the power of your mind that actually effects the changes that reduce the tension in your body. Eventually, when you have practiced your visualization technique sufficiently, you will be able to reduce muscle tension without being attached to the machine.

THE RELAXATION RESPONSE

Just as stress produces a variety of specific changes in the body, so, too, does deep relaxation. Dr. Herbert Benson of Harvard Medical School has called these physical changes "the relaxation response." They include slower breathing and heart rate, a lower blood pressure, and an improvement in digestion and circulation.

But what brings about this relaxation response? Dr. Benson believes that it is due to the brain's increased production of the large, slow alpha waves (see page 43), which occur after meditation. These replace the shorter, faster beta waves that are produced by the "active" brain. Alpha waves allow the brain to quiet down and possibly become more receptive to communications between its left and right hemispheres, which some theoreticians believe is essential for creative thinking.

Connected with these physical changes, which return the body to its natural balance, are changes in the mind and emotions. Apart from feeling calmer and more composed, your concentration and memory improve,

---

TRANQUILLITY THROUGH SENSORY DEPRIVATION

One way to quell the unrelenting stimulation of the modern world is to engage in a few minutes of sensory deprivation. In the past, floatation tanks were used. The tank was a large box that, when shut, did not

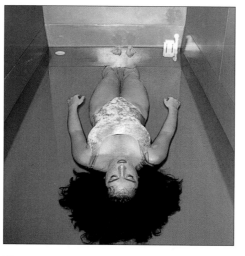

FLOATATION TANK
Spending half an hour in a floatation tank would relieve your cares. Isolated from all intrusions, you could relax in utter peace.

admit any light. In the bottom was enough water to fill about three bathtubs. The water was highly salted so that you would float easily. The absence of all types of stimuli and the gentle sensation of floating effortlessly in the water combined to make this a wonderfully relaxing experience.

Because of concerns about sanitation, however, most health spas have replaced floatation tanks with sensory deprivation devices. Here a person lies on a special water-filled mattress in a darkened, enclosed space for 10 to 20 minutes. The lack of sensory stimulation promotes deep relaxation.

Sensory deprivation is a good treatment for a number of stress-related illnesses and conditions. These include:

▶ *High blood pressure*

▶ *Migraines*

▶ *Headaches*

▶ *Persistent anxiety*

▶ *Muscle tension and fatigue*

you feel more resilient mentally, your mood lifts, and you are better able to put your difficulties into perspective. Because you are able to think more clearly, you will be able to assess situations better and find solutions to problems more easily.

VISUALIZATION

The brain is a very powerful organ. Just by thinking, you can either increase feelings of stress or reduce them. This is because the subconscious mind cannot tell the difference between a real experience and an imagined one. For example, having a near accident in your car will bring on such symptoms of stress as a racing pulse and churning stomach. These reactions will also occur if you vividly imagine a car crash. Lying in the sun on a peaceful balcony overlooking a deep blue sea will relax most people, but so will visualizing it.

In addition, visualization can help you meet difficult situations. This use of visualization is based on the principle that it is easier to do things when you have done them before. Thus, by vividly imagining the procedures that you are going to follow when you begin a new task, when you do finally tackle it you will proceed with much more confidence.

Visualization is especially effective in athletic endeavors. It has been shown that people, after learning the basics of a sport such as golf, perform better at the game if they have spent time visualizing the necessary movements or strokes than do players who have not done so. Professional athletes who spend time visualizing perfect performances as part of their training are finding that their performances do indeed improve.

Mental preparation

A great many potentially stressful situations can be eased by visualization. For example, if the thought of attending a party on the weekend makes you feel very nervous or anxious, then begin the week by imagining that you are watching some other guest at the gathering. Picture that person chatting away happily with the other guests and moving about confidently. Think about this image as often as you can over the next couple of days.

Now imagine yourself as the person you visualized, but still remain on the outside looking in—watch yourself having a good time. Let this image run through your mind as frequently as possible over the few days prior to the gathering. Then put yourself fully into your imagined scenario. Be that person who is conversing and socializing happily and confidently, and keep this thought uppermost in your mind right up to the time of the party. Once you get there, you may be surprised at how easy it is to mingle with the guests and enjoy yourself— but then you've done it all before!

Can I do it?

People often think that they will be unable to produce any mental pictures, claiming that they have no imagination whatsoever. These self-doubts are quite frequently caused by a misconception of what a mental image is supposed to be. Individuals believe that they should "see," with their eyes closed, a picture that exactly mirrors the images that they see with their eyes open. Although some people can indeed produce very powerful mental images, it is not essential to be able to do this for visualization to work for you.

Everyone is capable of visualizing. For example, if you have to describe your bedroom to an acquaintance, you will bring it to mind, perhaps internally focusing on particular features—the quilt on your bed, your rocking chair, or your wallpaper or curtains. You may even narrow your eyes while staring at a spot on the opposite wall—trying to "see" a pattern clearly, or you may use your hands to indicate a particular size or shape or texture to help you visualize more effectively.

Accessing pictures from your memory is very common in everyday life. In fact, you probably haven't realized that you have used the act of visualization hundreds of times in the past.

Music and soothing sounds can be great aids to visualization. Certain sounds on their own—the gentle noises of the rain forest, or the ocean lapping at the shore, or the wind in the trees—are often sufficient to ease tensions and evoke peaceful visual images, which can calm you completely. Today, listening to "new age" music, which is noted for its soothing melodies and instrumentals, has become an extremely popular form of relaxation, as are affirmation or subliminal tapes in which positive words and phrases are repeated.

Soothing sounds
Effective relaxation can be aided by appropriate background music. This is especially suitable when visualization is being used to unwind from a hectic and stressful day. You can choose from a range of commercially available audio tapes that provide a wide assortment of background effects.

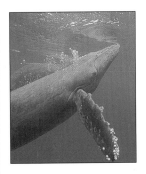

DEEP RELAXATION
Some people find that listening to the beautiful and haunting sounds of a whale song mentally transports them to the stress-free shores of the ocean.

Meditation

The simple act of concentrating the mind on a single word or object has been found to slow down body processes and increase serenity. People who meditate regularly find that their stress levels are greatly reduced.

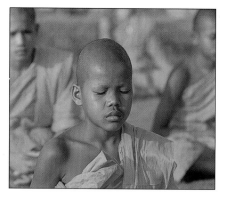

BUDDHIST MONK MEDITATING
Proponents of Buddhism incorporate meditation into their worship.

MEDITATION TEACHER WITH PUPIL
Your teacher will help you choose a mantra, and answer your questions.

For thousands of years, meditation has been part of many religions, including Buddhism and Hinduism. The most commonly used method in the West, transcendental meditation (TM), however, is of very recent origin. The Indian guru, Maharishi Mahesh Yogi, adapted the meditation techniques and postures of classic yoga to make them more accessible to modern, industrialized populations. TM was introduced to the West in 1959, and by the 1970's about 50,000 Americans were attending courses all across the United States.

How do you meditate?

Although there are numerous variations, the basic process in meditation is to concentrate for at least 15 minutes on a single word, thought, or object in order to rid your mind of all other thoughts and feelings. As this happens, the mind becomes increasingly focused until you reach a particular level of awareness, which has been described as a state of restful alertness.

What do you concentrate on?

A word or phrase, often known by the Sanskrit term *mantra*, is repeated over and over again. The mantra is frequently just a simple, single syllable word, such as peace, calm, or the Sanskrit *om*.

Another method is to concentrate on an object, such as a candle flame or a crystal, to help you purge your mind of any distracting thoughts.

How does meditation relieve stress?

Meditation produces a state of very deep relaxation. Your heart rate slows down, your level of oxygen consumption decreases, and after habitual practice your blood pressure will lower. Through meditation, your mind will become calmer, which will enable you to cope more effectively with the tensions of everyday life.

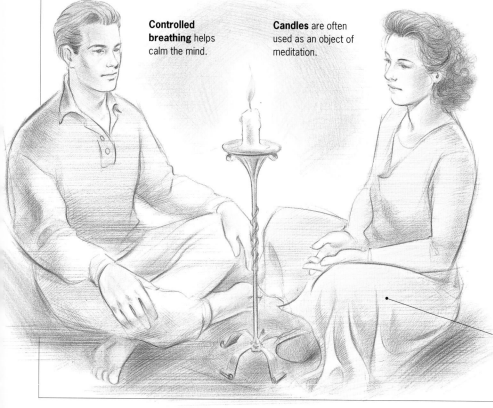

Controlled breathing helps calm the mind.

Candles are often used as an object of meditation.

Sitting cross-legged may not be comfortable for everyone. Find your own position, such as sitting on a chair.

Can I learn meditation by myself?

Yes, there are a number of books available on the subject; ideally, however, the correct posture and breathing techniques should be learned from a qualified teacher.

Who can teach me meditation?

Meditation is usually taught by people who have studied its techniques for many years. Teachers of TM complete a year-long training course; they are then registered with their country's national office.

What happens in a session?

First, your teacher will show you how to adopt the correct posture for meditating: sitting with legs crossed and back straight. Next you will be told to concentrate on breathing slowly and rhythmically. Then you will start to repeat your chosen mantra with your eyes closed, or you might be asked to partly close your eyes and fix them on a spot on the floor or a candle flame.

While repeating your mantra you will begin to empty your mind of all nagging concerns and tensions and let the word or object fill your consciousness. If any distracting noises or inner thoughts arise, you should immediately return to concentrating on your mantra. There is no need to fight distractions, just be passively aware of them, and gently bring your mind back to the object of your meditation. Initially, you will be asked to try to meditate for about 10 minutes. Although experienced individuals practice for much longer periods—ranging from 20 minutes to days, most beginners are amazed at how much their minds wander and how long 10 minutes can seem.

How long does it take to learn how to meditate?

Learning the basics typically should take only four sessions, with each session lasting about two hours, although the number will vary from teacher to teacher. After this, follow-up sessions may be given to see whether your meditation technique can be improved upon in any way. They also provide an opportunity for you to discuss any problems you have experienced with your teacher.

How does meditation differ from self-hypnosis?

The two techniques are very similar in that they both require a person to concentrate on an outside object or phrase to bring about a different level of consciousness. Self-hypnosis, however, usually has a specific goal in mind, and is a very good tool for reducing levels of stress or giving up smoking. Meditation is much more open-ended, because it helps people to achieve long-term, general physical and mental well-being.

Origins

Meditation is an ancient Eastern practice that may have originated with shamans and witch doctors in order to achieve a trance. In this way these early Asian tribesmen thought they could communicate with the spiritual world. Later, mantras and yoga poses were introduced as aids to meditation.

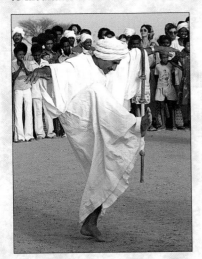

WHIRLING DERVISH
Muslim ascetics achieve, through rhythmic dance, a state of higher consciousness that is quite similar to meditation.

BRAIN WAVES

In different states of awareness the brain displays characteristic types of electrical activity. This electrical output can be recorded in wave patterns. Meditation has been shown to slow down the fast beta waves that are characteristic of a busy working day, and to help maintain more alpha waves, which are associated with feelings of calm and relaxation.

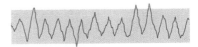

Alpha Waves (8–13 Hz)
Normal, calm state of mind.

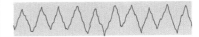

Beta Waves (14–30 Hz)
Active, busy state of mind.

Theta Waves (4–7 Hz)
Drowsiness.

DEDUCING STATE OF MIND
Your mental state can be determined from your brain wave patterns.

WHAT YOU CAN DO AT HOME

You don't need special training to meditate, but it is important to have an idea of the basic technique. You can begin now by choosing a word or a short sentence or statement, such as "I will succeed," or "I have unlimited potential." Take time each day (the first thing in the morning is best) to wordlessly repeat your phrase over and over for at least 10 minutes. Make sure you are sitting or reclining comfortably; close your eyes. While focusing on your word or phrase, breathe deeply and slowly; when distracting thoughts come, return to your word or phrase.

POSITIVE THINKING

You may not be able to change the weather or your job, but by changing the way you think, you can turn a negative experience into a positive one.

The philosophy of positivism

The French pharmacist Emile Coué (1857–1926) became famous for his belief that it's possible to teach our subconscious minds to be more positive. To do this we have to clear our minds of negative thoughts through repeating the positive phrase: "Every day in every way, I am getting better and better."

Coué's philosophy was expanded by Dr. Norman Vincent Peale (1898–1955), a Protestant minister in New York, who advised that anything is achievable if you have faith in yourself and refuse to accept the possibility of failure. His book, *The Power of Positive Thinking* (1952), is still in print and has sold over 20 million copies worldwide.

HOW FULL?
Positive thinkers would see this glass as half full, pessimists as half empty.

You can use your brain as a tool to help reduce stress. Positive thinking, also known as autosuggestion, can help you look at potentially stress-filled situations in a new light. For example, in the past, a teacher may have repeatedly told you that you were stupid. This information entered your subconscious, together with hurt and helpless feelings. Now, when you are older, perhaps your boss draws your attention to a mistake you have made. You are upset about this because it awakens childhood memories of being told you were inadequate. You then decide that you really must be incompetent. But the more you think about it—imagining your boss enjoying your discomfort or even laughing behind your back—the angrier you become. Your frustration, depression, and anger all add up to increased stress.

You could, however, break out of the straitjacket of the past by deciding to find a new way of seeing things. Instead of believing that your boss enjoys upsetting you, try to accept his or her comments as constructive criticism, whose purpose is to help you to increase your professionalism. This will make you feel that you and your boss are on the same side, and in the future you will be able to ask for help, thereby avoiding further mistakes. It may be hard at first to make yourself believe these positive thoughts, but with practice you will find yourself approaching life and all its problems and crises with more optimism and less stress.

A NEW LOOK AT LIFE

Another way to develop a positive attitude (and so decrease stress) is to make a point of noticing the good things that happen to you. Then take them into your subconscious by sending yourself positive messages—for instance, "I did that job very well." "I am perfectly capable of tackling that task." or "This person likes me." Once you begin talking to yourself in more positive terms, you will notice an improvement in your self-esteem and your performance.

Just avoiding negative thoughts and vocabulary when thinking about yourself can go a long way toward making you feel good and raising your self-esteem. Rather than believing that you are ignorant about a certain subject, tell yourself that you are capable of finding information about it if necessary. If someone unjustifiably accuses you of being aggressive, remember you have the right to be assertive (see page 72). Try substituting words such as challenging for impossible, opportunity for risk, fallible for incompetent, and exciting for dangerous.

Keep reversals of fortune in perspective, and try to see some of them as minor setbacks rather than major disasters. If you feel buried under an impossible workload, view it as a challenge you can learn from, but resolve not to let the situation continue for longer than is reasonable.

Future success

Thinking positively can be taken one step further to improve your performance in events or situations. Just as athletes use positive visualization to help them when they compete to run faster or jump higher, you, too, can use your newfound strength of mind to prepare for potentially stressful occasions such as a job interview, an examination, returning faulty goods to a supplier, or giving a speech. Facing any confrontation is always less traumatic when you are prepared. If you feel confident, you will be more in control, and your actions and words will be noticed. Soon others will comment on how you always seem to remain calm during a crisis or when making difficult and stressful decisions.

CHAPTER 3

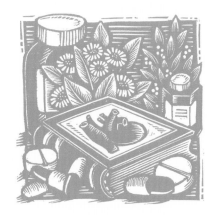

STRESS-RELATED DISEASES

---

*Research shows that too much stress
is a key factor in a wide variety of illnesses. In
fact, more than half of the ailments that are treated
in doctors' offices have some connection to stress.
Many alternative therapies are based on the link
between our emotional state and our physical well-
being. The ones offered in this chapter provide
a wide range of healing remedies to ease
stress and return you to health.*

STRESS AND HEALTH

Medical evidence confirms that stress influences the immune system. Be aware of the role of stress in various ailments and you may be able to guard your health more effectively.

For centuries the theory that too much or prolonged stress can cause disease and aggravate existing conditions has been just that—a theory. While doctors had a great deal of anecdotal evidence to support a cause-and-effect connection between stress and illness, there was little actual scientific proof. But circumstances changed dramatically in the early 1970's when neuroscientists unraveled the way the brain transmits messages. What they saw revolutionized how we think about the brain. They knew that the brain had an intricate system of communications that relied on natural chemicals, known as neurotransmitters, to act as a kind of chemical bridge, sending and receiving information from one brain cell to another. What they didn't know was how these neurotransmitters worked. Thanks to dogged research, they discovered that certain neurotransmitters connected to specific sites in the brain with a lock and key system. This explained why the pain-killing drug morphine, for instance, is effective against pain—it bonds to particular receptor sites in the brain that relieve pain.

Further study soon revealed that under special circumstances, such as prolonged physical stress caused by long-distance running or childbirth, the brain manufactures its own morphine-like substances, known as endorphins, that bond to the same pain-relieving receptors.

If the brain had the ability to relieve pain, what about other emotions? This question was answered by the discovery of the function behind other neurotransmitters such as serotonin and dopamine. Low levels of serotonin, for instance, were found in people with severe depression; diminished amounts of serotonin and dopamine were found in those suffering from anxiety. The impact of these neurotransmitters on the emotions has spawned new drugs to treat depression, such as fluoxetine (Prozac), which affects the level of serotonin in the brain.

New research, however, now shows that the receptors for these neurotransmitters are found not just in the brain but also in the digestive track and the immune system—the lymph nodes, the thymus gland, bone marrow, the spleen, and specialized lymphocytes.

To a number of researchers, this startling discovery suggests that the immune system must be connected to the nervous system,

STRESS HITS WHERE IT HURTS

From migraine to irritable bowel syndrome, stress causes a wide range of ailments. The suppression of the immune system when you are under pressure can also make you more vulnerable to infectious diseases such as colds and flu.

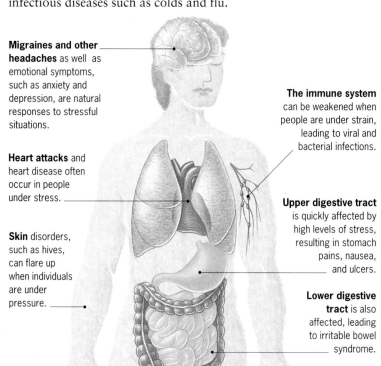

Migraines and other headaches as well as emotional symptoms, such as anxiety and depression, are natural responses to stressful situations.

Heart attacks and heart disease often occur in people under stress.

Skin disorders, such as hives, can flare up when individuals are under pressure.

The immune system can be weakened when people are under strain, leading to viral and bacterial infections.

Upper digestive tract is quickly affected by high levels of stress, resulting in stomach pains, nausea, and ulcers.

Lower digestive tract is also affected, leading to irritable bowel syndrome.

and that fear and anxiety, two common emotions associated with stress, have a direct impact on the immune system. Others, however, feel that stress and the associated emotions are too varied and complex for us to make a direct connection between emotions and illness. Nevertheless, enough scientific indicators point in this direction that many health care practitioners are urging people to use stress management techniques to prevent illness and promote health.

Many alternative therapists have long recognized the mind-body link. Thus their approach is to treat a person's mental and emotional state as well as physical condition. They do this by relieving the stress along with its physical manifestations. Their success has encouraged orthodox physicians to take a new look at the role of stress in disease and in many cases has helped to transform the way they treat their patients.

STRESS REACTIONS

Numerous studies have tried to pin down the role of stress in disease. Researchers know that when a person is under stress, the entire body is affected. The heart beats faster and more forcibly, blood pressure rises, stores of fatty acids and glucose are released into the bloodstream, and the bronchioles (breathing tubes) in the lungs expand to let in more air. Certain blood vessels dilate and others constrict to divert blood to where it is most needed. The blood also becomes stickier to encourage clots to form so that bleeding will be reduced if any injury occurs. There are other changes as well, such as an increase in stomach acids, reduction in the production of saliva, and an increase in the urge to urinate.

The stress response also calls for the immediate suppression of the immune system. The stress hormones, adrenaline and noradrenaline, act to inhibit the way white blood cells (which are part of the immune system) respond to bacteria, viruses, and cancer cells. Usually the suppression of the immune system is not harmful and once the stress has passed, all the body systems return to normal.

Long-term stress, however, can result in many health problems: heart disease high blood pressure hypertension, hormonal disorders, backache, and migraine. It also aggravates disorders connected with the immune system, such as allergies and asthma.

Heart and circulatory problems

A specialist in heart disease at London's Charing Cross Hospital, Dr. Peter Nixon, has described what he calls the human function curve (see below). This shows what happens when stress makes people attempt increasingly demanding tasks beyond the point at which they are either physically or mentally capable of carrying them out.

Here is how it works: as the body copes with physical exertion and minor stress, it is normal to have peaks of raised blood pressure. The chemicals secreted by the body in these circumstances cause the arteries to constrict, so that their diameter is reduced. This means that pressure must be increased to keep the blood going through the circulatory system.

High blood pressure (hypertension) refers to a consistent measurement that is greater than 140/90. If blood pressure levels are very high—or have been elevated for a long time—the arterial walls become more rigid and prone to damage, and there is an increased risk for kidney disease and stroke.

In addition, hormones released during stress break down the body's fat stores in order to provide more fuel for energy requirements. As a result, levels of fatty acids and other lipids in the blood increase, contributing to fatty deposits inside the arterial walls, which gradually block the blood flow. This can lead to coronary heart disease in susceptible individuals, especially those with diets high in saturated fat who may already have coronary artery clogging.

Heart disease: the international view

The incidence of heart disease varies across the world. It is high in the UK, U.S., and Eastern Europe, while in Mediterranean countries it is strikingly low. In the UK and U.S., a diet high in saturated fat has been implicated, and so have high levels of stress among the general population. This is partly due to a faster and more pressured pace of life. In the Mediterranean countries, the lifestyle is slower. Moreover, the diet is high in olive oil, a monounsaturated fat, and red wine—both of which appear to protect the heart against disease.

THE HUMAN FUNCTION CURVE
The first part of the blue curve shows how performance improves while a person is under stress. The second part represents what individuals believe they are capable of while stress continues. The red curve, which drops sharply, reflects what actually happens—diminished capability and impaired health.

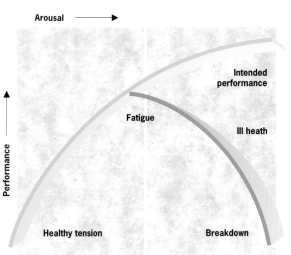

Arousal

Intended performance

Fatigue

Ill heath

Performance

Healthy tension

Breakdown

Getting away from it all

Going to a retreat for a few days, or even a week, is an option for stressed-out souls who seek calm, spiritual contemplation, or simply some rest and recuperation. In the United States, it is estimated that 3 million people go to some form of a retreat every week.

Retreats have been organized by Buddhist centers, convents, monasteries, yoga healing centers, and New Age groups. Each offers an individual approach to help people refresh their lives, from days of silence and/or prayer, to one-on-one counseling, to chanting, dancing, and walking. Most retreats are fairly inexpensive and make a novel vacation from the stress of everyday life.

Digestive disorders

Some of the most common symptoms of stress are pains in the stomach, indigestion, heartburn, and nausea. Irritable bowel syndrome—a chronic malfunction of the intestines that causes abdominal pain, diarrhea or constipation, and heartburn—can also be caused by high anxiety levels, and it worsens when sufferers are under pressure.

While stress may be the culprit behind many ailments, it should not rule out other factors. A case in point are ulcers. Doctors once believed they were caused solely by stress. New research reveals that most peptic ulcers are the result of a common bacterial infection. Once the bacteria in question, *helicobacter pylori*, are treated with antibiotics and antacids, peptic ulcers clear up. However, an interesting question remains. Since most adults harbor *helicobacter pylori*, why are so few afflicted with ulcers? The answer, to date, is that stress contributes to peptic ulcers by lowering the immune system's defenses against the bacteria.

Reproductive problems

While anxiety depresses the sex drive in both men and women, it can also have a direct effect on fertility. Studies of male fertility show that emotional stress, such as the kind caused by the death of a loved one, can reduce sperm count by 12 percent.

Stress can also play havoc with a woman's menstrual cycle. Menstrual irregularity, which can have a number of causes, is often related to increased stress. Moreover, stress can precipitate "spontaneous" abortions and premature labor.

Allergies, asthma, and skin disorders

An allergy is the severe reaction of the body's immune system to various substances, such as pollen or dust, that are usually harmless. Responses can vary widely, but sneezing and watery eyes are common.

Asthma—another disease that often has an allergic component—is thought to be affected by stress, but the attacks cause anxiety in themselves, and the reaction is hard to separate from the trigger. In one investigation, however, the asthma of 70 percent of the sufferers under scrutiny had a significant emotional component.

Many skin problems are exacerbated when the sufferer is under pressure. Such complaints include hives (urticaria), which can flare up in direct response to stress. Psoriasis, which occurs irregularly, can erupt when stress levels are high, as can acne, neurodermatitis, and persistent hair pulling (or trichitillomania). People with allergic eczema often find their condition worsens when they are stressed.

Treatment for stress-related illness

Unlike modern Western medicine, which targets a specific problem, alternative remedies are holistic in nature. That is, they aim to treat the whole person, physically, mentally, and, in some cases, spiritually, in order to restore the body to a state of balance so it is able to successfully withstand disease.

Alternative medicine presents a unique approach to the problem of stress because it attempts to address the cause of the stress as well as the physical manifestation of disease and illness. Thus, alternative practitioners typically ask a great many more questions concerning their patients' quality of life than Western doctors would. This is so that they can accurately identify the underlying causes of the symptoms. In that way these therapists are looking to provide "whole health" to sufferers.

Alternative therapies consist of a variety of different approaches to the body—and what ails it and cures it. A number of these therapies, such as acupuncture, acupressure, and homeopathy, work on the principle that disease is due to various imbalances in the body; if balances are restored, the body's ability to combat disease is strengthened, and its capacity to heal itself renewed. In terms of stress this may mean a reduction in depression, a lowering of blood pressure, the promotion of calming sleep, and deep relaxation.

Other techniques, such as the Alexander Technique, osteopathy, chiropractic, and massage, concentrate on reducing tension and relieving pain that was caused by stress, either through physical manipulation or by the correction of poor posture.

Eastern practices, including yoga, tai chi, and meditation, emphasize the power of the mind in overcoming the sources of stress and teach their followers ways of harnessing their mental energy to maintain health.

Finally therapies, like aromatherapy, are and especially suited to self-care, use oils to aid relaxation.

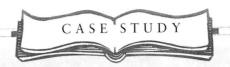
Working Up to an Illness

Persistent anxiety can lead to physical discomforts or to real illness. Minor ailments, like indigestion, may not be life-threatening, but can cause misery, whereas major stress disorders like hypertension can be dangerous. For these reasons we must recognize signs, such as irritability and sleeplessness, that tell us we are under pressure, and take steps to prevent serious consequences.

Philip, a 45-year-old social worker, puts in long hours. Manpower shortages have forced more cases onto his workload, and he is finding it hard to complete all his duties. His long hours at the office leave little time to be with his wife, Judy, and when they do meet he is irritable and tired. He has had several bouts of heart palpitations and suffers extreme fatigue. Philip feels overwhelmed by his work, yet he feels powerless to do anything about it.

One morning, Judy is shocked to find Philip sitting in his car having palpitations before an important meeting at work. He tells her he is terrified he might die during these attacks, and is afraid he could have a serious heart problem.

WHAT PHILIP SHOULD DO

Rather than pushing himself beyond the limit of endurance, Philip needs to share his concerns with others. First, he should find out whether his health is as bad as he fears. If tests prove he has a heart problem, he will have to take steps to protect himself from a possible heart attack. If his concerns are groundless, he will need to think about the causes of his symptoms and look for ways of alleviating them. Counseling would help Philip work through any unresolved emotional issues.

Philip also needs to consider his marriage. His irritability is driving Judy away. If he wants her continued support, he must become aware of how his work is affecting his relationship with her.

Action Plan

HEALTH
Visit a doctor for a checkup. Find out what therapies may help to keep heart disease at bay. Make sure that his diet is healthy.

PARTNERS
Reopen lines of communication with Judy to air problems. Suggest a vacation together.

WORK
Discuss with colleagues ways of alleviating work pressures. Arrange a meeting with boss and suggest that some of his duties be delegated, at least for the short term.

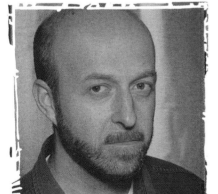

HEALTH
Stress at work can manifest itself in a wide range of both physical and emotional symptoms.

PARTNERS
Workaholics often have little to give their personal relationships. This can lead to marriage breakdown.

WORK
Overwork causes many unpleasant symptoms and can make people resentful of their employer.

HOW THINGS TURNED OUT FOR PHILIP

Philip's cardiogram and other tests were normal, but he does have high blood pressure (hypertension). The doctor explains that it is due to stress, and suggests he exercise and learn some relaxation techniques. Philip takes this advice, and begins running a mile a day and signs up for a class on meditation. He tells his boss that his excessive workload is affecting his health, and his boss agrees to lessen his caseload. His blood pressure soon returns to normal, and the panic attacks disappear.

Homeopathy

Homeopathy is a system of medicine that uses highly diluted substances to boost the body's natural ability to cure itself. Practitioners view illness as a sign of inner imbalance and consider all aspects of patients' lives when treating complaints.

DEADLY NIGHTSHADE (BELLADONNA)
Tiny doses of both the flowers and berries of this poisonous plant are used by homeopaths to treat stress-related headaches, particularly those that produce throbbing pain.

Homeopaths define illness differently than conventional physicians. They believe that the symptoms of an illness are signs of how the body is attempting to cure itself, and their efforts are directed toward enhancing those efforts. To do this, they prescribe substances that induce similar symptoms when given to healthy people in large amounts. This is called treating "like with like" (*homoios* is Greek for "like"). Practitioners use a holistic approach, considering the psychological as well as the physical needs of their patients, and tailor remedies to the individual.

Origins

Homeopathic medicine was founded as a discipline in the 18th century by the German physician Samuel Hahnemann (1755–1843).

Hahnemann experimented on himself with a malaria remedy called cinchona bark. He took the medicine and experienced malaria-like symptoms, even though he was healthy. He wondered if other medicines also produced the symptoms of an illness in a healthy person but relieved them in someone who was sick, and he began to investigate this possibility.

In 1811, the *Homoeopathic Materia Medica* was published, in which Hahnemann described his theories, as well as giving a list of remedies. His ideas gained approval, and homeopathy spread to France,

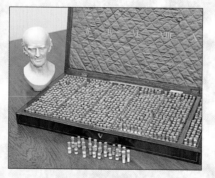

HAHNEMANN'S REMEDIES
Hahnemann's own medical kit, containing around 200 bottles of homeopathic medicines, can be seen in the National Museum of American History, Washington, D.C.

then to Great Britain and the United States. Homeopathy was supplanted by other medical therapies in early 20th-century America, but it is regaining popularity as a helpful adjunct to conventional medicine.

What are homeopathic remedies made from?
Most are based on extracts from minerals, plants, and animals. A number have long-established histories of medicinal use, including those that are derived from poisons. For instance, physicians and homeopaths use foxglove (*Digitalis purpurea*) as a medicine—digitalis.

How are homeopathic medicines prepared?
First, the beneficial substance is soaked in either alcohol or water to form a tincture. Next, a drop of the tincture is added to a vial of water in a ratio of 1:10 or 1:100 (1 drop of tincture to 9 or 99 drops of water). Finally, the vial is shaken. This procedure is repeated until an effective potency is achieved. The remedies are sold as liquids or as pills.

How dilute are homeopathic medicines?
No trace of the original beneficial substance can actually be found in the remedies. It is thought that, despite this, the medicines have imprinted themselves on the molecular structure of the liquid they were diluted with, and somehow remain effective.

If nothing remains of the original substance, how can it treat illness?
Homeopaths believe that the more dilute a remedy, the more powerful it is. They ascribe its effectiveness to the transmission of "vital energy"

that resonates within the patient's body. This benefit is imparted to the remedy by the mixture being shaken vigorously, or "succussed," after each dilution. Substances that are diluted without shaking do not work.

How do homeopaths treat patients?

Homeopaths take a detailed history of the patient, including personal circumstances, general health, and the medical aspects of the complaint. They will also ask a wide range of questions so that they can build up a comprehensive psychological profile. The homeopath will then prescribe a remedy tailored to the particular patient. As a result of this individualized treatment, people with the same illness may be given quite different medicines. Homeopaths may

THERAPIST WITH PATIENT
In the first consultation, the homeopath will ask questions about your medical history, energy level, sleep patterns and food preferences.

prescribe different remedies, or the same remedy at different potencies, in subsequent consultations. The aim is to cure each "layer" of disorders until the central, underlying condition is resolved.

How is homeopathy effective in treating stress?

Homeopaths take a two-pronged approach. If stress is the underlying disorder, they will prescribe remedies to deal with the specific symptoms, and may suggest changes in their patients' lives that can help them tackle the underlying causes of their anxiety.Homeopaths spend a great deal of time talking to their patients, who may derive psychological benefit from this. Homeopathy has a good success rate with people whose

Patients find it very therapeutic to discuss their problems.

problems—such as migraine headaches or irritable bowel syndrome—often have an emotional or psychological component.

How quickly does homeopathic treatment take effect?

Serious treatment may require several stages with at least four to six weeks between visits. Symptoms may worsen for a time. This is known as "a healing crisis" and is a good sign, so long as the reaction is not too severe, because it shows that the treatment is stimulating the body to heal itself.

How do I find a homeopath?

Contact The National Center for Homeopathy at 801 North Fairfax Street, Alexandria, Virginia 22314. For a nominal fee they will send you a directory that lists reputable homeopaths in your area.

WHAT YOU CAN DO AT HOME

Once you have your homeopathic remedy there are a few simple rules that should be followed. Store all remedies in a cool, dry place. To maintain their potency, remedies must never be handled, allowed to come into contact with any strong scent, or transferred into a container that previously held any other remedy. Don't drink coffee and alcohol during the course of treatment; some homeopaths may also ask you not to eat peppermint or use mint-flavored toothpaste.

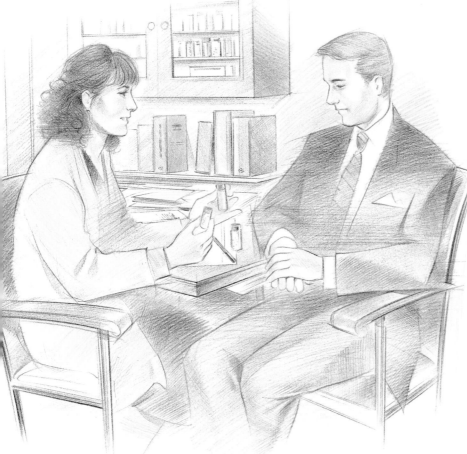

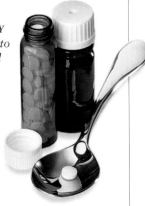

TAKING A REMEDY
Tip the remedy onto a clean spoon, and place it in your mouth. Suck it or allow it to dissolve under your tongue; do not swallow it whole.

Chiropractic

Stress-related tension can cause nerve compression, which in turn may induce head, neck, and back pain. To relieve it, chiropractors apply manual pressure to muscles, bones, and joints, particularly the spine.

7 cervical vertebrae

12 thoracic vertebrae

5 lumbar vertebrae

Sacrum

Coccyx

THE STRAIN ON THE SPINE
Powerful muscles attached to the spine contract as the body moves, sometimes pulling heavily on the spine. Many backaches stem from strain and tension in these muscles, and disappear quickly when the stress is relieved.

The word *chiropractic* (from the Greek words *cheiro* and *prakrikos*) means "done by hand." The principle behind chiropractic is that misalignments, often called subluxations, of the vertebrae can impinge on the spinal nerves and cause pain and illness.

If a nerve is pinched, pain can occur at any point along its path. Pain that occurs away from the site of the entrapment is called referred pain. For example, the sciatic nerve extends from the base of the spine to the foot. If it is pinched near the spine, there may be pain in the lower back, the knee, or toes.

Stress is a particularly insidious factor in many ailments because it can cause pain, which in turn can lead to muscle spasm, causing more stress, and so on. Chiropractic treatment can help relieve muscle spasm and disrupt this cycle.

How does a chiropractor make a diagnosis?

At the consultation, a chiropractor will ask the patient about family medical history, recent stressful events, and habits and diet. He will then make a visual and manual examination of the patient, looking for signs of injury, bad posture,

Origins

Chiropractic was founded in 1895, by Daniel David Palmer (1845–1913), a Canadian healer who practiced in Iowa. Before he developed his own system of manipulation, Palmer had learned osteopathy, an earlier practice which had been established in Missouri by Dr. Andrew Taylor Still and involved less vigorous manipulation of the spine.

Palmer's first success was with a deaf man who claimed that his affliction was due to a back injury. Physical examination revealed that the man had a misaligned vertebra, which Palmer manipulated back into place, thereby restoring the man's hearing. After this, Palmer formulated a theory that all living things have an "innate intelligence" that flows through the central nervous system and regulates all its vital functions. He developed treatments to free this intelligence from interference and allow it to flow freely in the body.

After Palmer died, it took another 50 years before chiropractic gained acceptance (and state licensing) throughout the United States. It is now the third largest primary health care system, with more than 40,000 practitioners worldwide.

As chiropractic grew, divisions began to appear within the practice. Some chiropractors began to use high-tech equipment such as x-ray and ultrasound machines, which others thought was a departure from Palmer's natural approach. The British founder of McTimoney chiropractic, John McTimoney (1914–1981), established

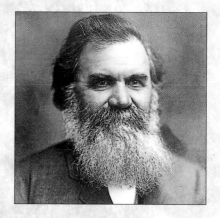

DANIEL DAVID PALMER
Modern chiropractic was founded by Daniel David Palmer. The treatment seeks to cure disorders through spinal manipulation.

his own school in Oxfordshire in 1972 to teach "pure" chiropractic, using no special equipment, no drugs, and usually no x-rays.

muscle spasm, tenderness, excessive or restricted limb movement, or displaced joints. Usually she will have x-rays taken before giving treatment.

Which disorders can be treated by a chiropractor?

Several stress-related ailments—for example, neuralgia, and certain rheumatic and arthritic disorders—can be relieved by chiropractic treatments, as can nonspecific neck and back pain. A chiropractic manipulation, more commonly called an adjustment, can help ease many of the symptoms of nerve compression such as tingling, numbness, or "pins and needles." To ease muscle spasms, some chiropractors apply heat packs to the affected area.

Is chiropractic treatment better for back pain than orthodox treatment?

A 1988 study of 20,000 back-injury cases in Florida found that subjects who chose chiropractic therapy returned to work in a third of the time compared with individuals who had chosen orthodox treatment (which included bed rest, physiotherapy, and pain-killers). However, in 1994, in a randomized trial of patients with low back pain, the Iowa Spine Research Center found that there was no significant difference in outcome between massage, chiropractic manipulation, and wearing a corset or brace.

Are there any disorders that chiropractic cannot treat?

Pain from fractures, infections, tumors, or arthritis that involves inflammation cannot be treated. Children should not undergo chiropractic manipulation.

Is chiropractic ever dangerous?

It can be dangerous in the hands of an unqualified person. Each of six different government inquiries worldwide, however, concluded that modern chiropractic therapy, when carried out by an adequately trained chiropractor, is safe. Be sure, however, to check with your doctor

before visiting the chiropractor, to find out if chiropractic treatment is contraindicated.

How is treatment carried out?

A combination of over 30 different adjustment techniques is used, most commonly a series of short, rapid, shallow thrusts. Chiropractors also employ heat therapy, ice packs, traction (in which a weight is attached

to part of the body to pull it into alignment), or ultrasound (in which very high sound waves penetrate the skin and the energy of the vibrations dissipates as heat).

Where can I find a chiropractor?

The World Chiropractic Alliance in Chandler, Arizona, provides referrals for chiropractors nationwide, and public information services.

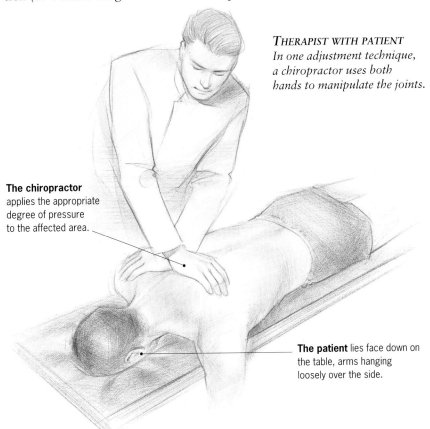

THERAPIST WITH PATIENT
In one adjustment technique, a chiropractor uses both hands to manipulate the joints.

The chiropractor applies the appropriate degree of pressure to the affected area.

The patient lies face down on the table, arms hanging loosely over the side.

WHAT YOU CAN DO AT HOME

A regular stretch of your shoulders will help keep your upper spine flexible, and release any tension you are holding there. Do the stretch slowly and smoothly whenever you can.

STEP ONE
Clasp your hands behind your back.

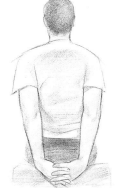

STEP TWO
Push your chest forward and up and stretch your arms back. Hold for a few seconds.

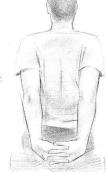

ANXIETY AND DEPRESSION

It is estimated that up to 30 percent of the Western world's population suffers periods of depression from too much pressure, and many more people suffer stress-related anxiety.

Some degree of anxiety and fear is a natural human response to a challenge. In the right circumstances they will help you spring into action. But constantly heightened levels of anxiety and fear can lead to physical as well as emotional problems, especially if they are caused by situations in which you are powerless, or have impossible schedules or deadlines you can't meet. For some people the anxiety may be external, such as living in a dangerous neighborhood. In such cases, the fear of violence and lack of control over it may lead to debilitating panic attacks or depression.

Anxiety and fear can also play a role in numerous physical complaints. Common symptoms include tension headaches, chest and neck pains, and backache. Sometimes, people with acute anxiety develop psychosomatic conditions that mimic the symptoms of an organic disease, for example, anxiety-caused chest pains that can feel like a heart attack.

Sometimes stress is so intense that it precipitates a panic attack. This is a brief period of acute anxiety, characterized by profuse sweating, light-headedness, palpitations, tightness in the chest, and a sinking feeling in the stomach. Panic attacks often happen without warning, though they are usually associated with a stressful event, such as a crowded elevator. It is also common to

SEX AND STRESS

Communication problems between partners can cause a great deal of anxiety. This releases stress hormones that counteract the effects of testosterone, the hormone responsible for sexual arousal. If this leads to impotence in a man, or to loss of sexual drive in a woman, tension will increase and sexual failure will then become yet another source of stress.

If you are experiencing a sexual problem you should visit your physician to discover if anything is physically wrong, or if any medication you are taking is responsible. If there is no physical cause, then ask yourself why you are feeling so anxious and talk it over with your partner. You could also try changing the times and places you make love. Plan for a vacation; the change of scene may

reawaken your interest in lovemaking. If the idea of intercourse worries you, simply touch and hug each other; touching in itself will relieve tension and may help to reestablish communication.

VICIOUS CYCLE: EFFECT OF STRESS ON DESIRE

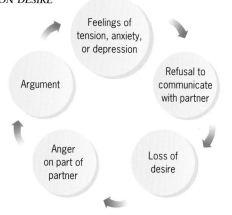

Feelings of tension, anxiety, or depression

Refusal to communicate with partner

Loss of desire

Anger on part of partner

Argument

hyperventilate, which upsets the balance of oxygen and carbon dioxide in the blood. If you feel an attack is imminent, breathe in and out of a paper bag to restore oxygen concentrations to normal. If a paper bag is not available, try simply holding your breath for as long as possible.

DEPRESSION

Everyone feels down occasionally, but the feeling usually passes. This is not the case with severe or clinical depression. Severe and long-lasting depression produces very specific physical symptoms, such as a loss (or occasionally, an increase) of appetite, difficulty in getting to sleep, and early morning waking. Other symptoms include constipation, extreme fatigue, and a general feeling of malaise.

It also produces mental and emotional symptoms. People with clinical depression often report a feeling of emptiness, a lack of interest in everything, and loss of energy. Food is tasteless, flowers odorless, meetings with friends and family joyless; in serious cases the sufferer is full of despair, loses hope in everything, and thinks of suicide. It is important that someone suffering from these symptoms seek medical help as soon as possible. Fortunately there are many treatments available, ranging from counseling to medication.

Causes of depression

Clinical depression falls into two categories. One is the reactive type—the emotional gloom is due to a person's response to a recent stressful event, such as a bereavement, the loss of a job, or divorce. This kind of depression usually gets better with time.

The second kind is known as endogenous depression. This illness has several forms, including manic-depression (also known as bipolar disease), unipolar depression, and postpartum depression.

There are many theories about the causes of depression. Hormonal imbalance—which is especially the case with new mothers suffering from postpartum depression—genetic factors, major stressful situations in the past that were never resolved, for instance, the death of a parent when one was a child, have all been implicated. There is evidence that depression is caused by an overwhelming accumulation of stress, which depletes the brain of serotonin (see page 46).

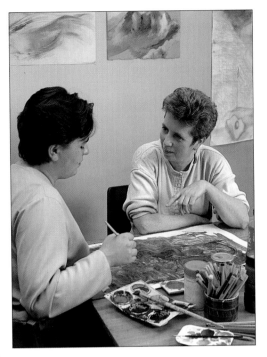

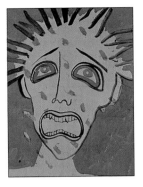

ART THERAPY
For people with stress-related psychological problems, art therapy (left) can release hidden feelings, such as the anger and frustration starkly exhibited in the above drawing.

Learned helplessness

One theory about depression has been put forward by the psychologist M. E. P. Seligman. Seligman gave electric shocks to caged animals who, when they tried to escape, found their ways barred. After a while, they began to show the symptoms of lethargy and listlessness typical of depression. Then Seligman gave the animals the same shocks but left open the cage doors. Although now free to leave, the animals stayed in the cages, having learned to be helpless. Seligman extended his theory of "learned helplessness" to human beings, and proposed that depression comes from people feeling powerless about their lives.

His ideas have been borne out in a study of workers in high-stress jobs, among them assembly-line operators under heavy pressure to perform but with little say about how they worked. The workers took more medicine for depression than their managers, who had more control over their lives.

continued on page 58

DID YOU KNOW?

Many famous historical figures have suffered from depression. One of the most notable was Sir Winston Churchill, the British statesman and prime minister, who called his attacks of incapacitating depression his "black dog."

Yoga

Yoga—the Sanskrit word for "union"—is an ancient Indian tradition that combines exercise and meditation. It is useful for relieving stress, and the stretching exercises are beneficial for everyone, regardless of age or level of fitness.

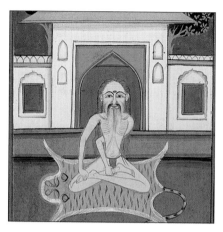

A VARIATION OF THE LOTUS POSITION
One of the classic yoga poses, this version is for advanced yoga students.

With its emphasis on gentle stretching and deep, even breathing, yoga postures are good for health in many ways. In particular, the exercises can help ease muscle tension, lower blood pressure, and calm nerves.

As with any attempt at behavior modification, yoga works best if practiced regularly. Practitioners advocate doing yoga exercised daily,

even if you do them for just 10 minutes, and even if these 10 minutes are taken in two- or three-minute sessions throughout the day.

Yoga's philosophy is noncompetitive and non-stressful. The intention is to make the sessions as pleasant as possible, so that you will be inspired to practice the movements and deep breathing regularly.

GENTLE YOGA EXERCISES

Pick a time when you will not be disturbed, and a space where you can move freely. Breathe naturally while holding a pose. Hold the pose for as long as is comfortable, then come slowly back to the starting position and repeat on the other side.

THE TRIANGLE POSE

Start with feet wide apart and parallel, toes turned slightly in, hips facing forward, and arms by your side.

Hand and wrist should be relaxed, with stretch coming from the armpit.

Shoulders should be down and relaxed.

Exhale slowly as you bend. Inhale slowly and deeply as you straighten up.

Hips face forward.

Stretch from the outside of your leg and up your side.

Weight should be balanced on both feet.

The hand may not reach this far down, but you will improve with practice.

1 *Turn your right foot out and raise your arms to shoulder height.*

2 *Stretch out slowly to the right. Do not let your body bend forward, but be careful to keep it in one plane.*

3 *Bend sideways toward your ankle, until your right hand reaches your leg; stretch your left arm straight up.*

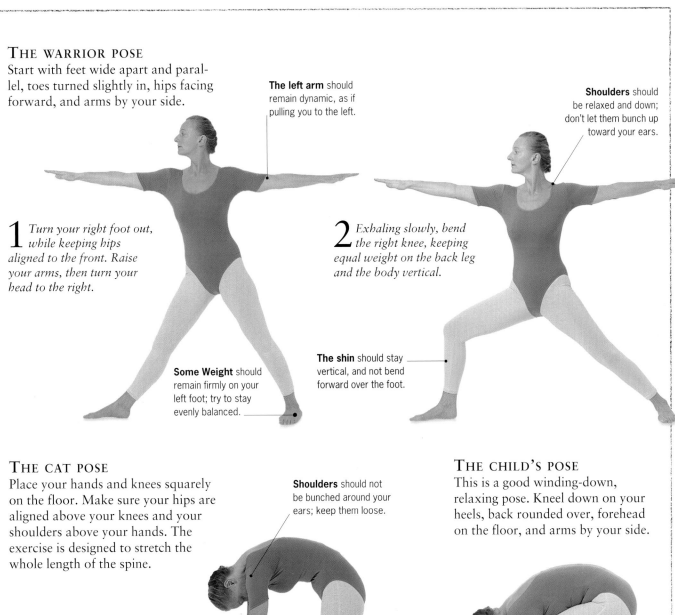

THE WARRIOR POSE

Start with feet wide apart and parallel, toes turned slightly in, hips facing forward, and arms by your side.

The left arm should remain dynamic, as if pulling you to the left.

Shoulders should be relaxed and down; don't let them bunch up toward your ears.

1 *Turn your right foot out, while keeping hips aligned to the front. Raise your arms, then turn your head to the right.*

2 *Exhaling slowly, bend the right knee, keeping equal weight on the back leg and the body vertical.*

Some Weight should remain firmly on your left foot; try to stay evenly balanced.

The shin should stay vertical, and not bend forward over the foot.

THE CAT POSE

Place your hands and knees squarely on the floor. Make sure your hips are aligned above your knees and your shoulders above your hands. The exercise is designed to stretch the whole length of the spine.

Shoulders should not be bunched around your ears; keep them loose.

THE CHILD'S POSE

This is a good winding-down, relaxing pose. Kneel down on your heels, back rounded over, forehead on the floor, and arms by your side.

Aim to stretch the upper part of your back, not just the lumbar region.

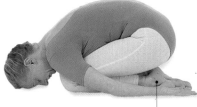

2 *Exhaling, round your back upward, letting your head drop down.*

Place a cushion over your heels if you cannot kneel all the way back on them. It is important to have a firm base from which to stretch forward.

Hands should be flat, and fingers stretched. The exercise will help to strengthen your wrists.

1 *Inhaling slowly, lift your head upward, stretching from your chest and arching your back.*

CAUTION

Before starting any exercise regimen, check with your physician, especially if you are pregnant or suffering from high blood pressure, a back injury, or a heart or breathing disorder.

COPING WITH DEPRESSION

Try one or more of the following "natural" remedies to ease the symptoms of depression.

▶ *Share your feelings with a trusted friend or relative, and enjoy the support and reassurance he or she can offer.*

▶ *Avoid spending too much time alone. Going out can introduce you to new activities and to people who may help your recovery.*

▶ *Increase your intake of fresh fruits and vegetables, and fish, lean meats, whole-grain cereals, and low-fat dairy products. A healthy diet will make you feel less lethargic.*

▶ *Eat lightly throughout the day instead of having a few large meals. This will steady your blood sugar levels and help prevent mood swings.*

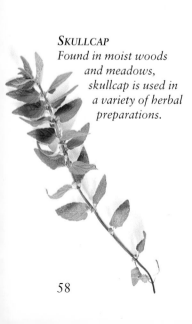

SKULLCAP
Found in moist woods and meadows, skullcap is used in a variety of herbal preparations.

To improve morale, some companies now give workers more decision-making power over their working procedures, and mix routine tasks and duties with new challenges.

TREATING ANXIETY AND DEPRESSION

Although anxiety and depression are common conditions, there is still a considerable stigma attached to them. Many people feel ashamed or embarrassed about admitting to emotional problems, even to their physicians. They worry that they will be regarded as weak or neurotic, and so they struggle on and refuse to seek help.

And yet, talking about your feelings to a friend or family member can help to ease mild anxiety or depression; indeed, just the act of unburdening yourself may help you feel remarkably better as you will be able to gain perspective on your feelings.

If you are suffering from depression-like symptoms, it might be worthwhile visiting your physician, who will try to determine if there are any underlying physical causes. If no physical illness is found and your condition warrants it, your doctor may prescribe a tranquillizer for anxiety or an anti-depressant for depression. Bear in mind, however, that long-term use of such medications can lead to dependence. While the newer class of antidepressants such as Prozac (fluoxe-

Pathways to health

Aromatherapy can be effective in helping to relieve anxiety and depression. Some essential oils used for this purpose have calming properties; others invigorate or lift the spirits. (See page 68 for how to use them.)

A massage using rosemary can help ease the rigidness and pain—so often brought on by tension and worry—in the muscles of the neck and shoulders. Just add a few drops of the essential oil to a base oil such as almond.

Lavender essential oil may calm those who are suffering from anxiety, and it will also promote restful sleep. Add a few drops of this oil to your bath, or place one to two drops on the edge of your pillow. Other calming essential oils include sandalwood, geranium, and clary sage.

tine) have proven effective for treating depression, they can cause side effects.

An herbal remedy that relieves moderate depression without side effects is St. John's wort (*Hypericum*), available as capsules, a tea, and a tincture. This herb is the leading treatment for depression in Germany. Studies have found that the optimum dosage is 300 mg of 0.3 percent of hypericin, the active ingredient, taken three times a day with food, to avoid stomach upset. Standardized capsules are best because you don't know how much active ingredient is contained in tea or other forms. (St. John's wort is not recommended during pregnancy and it makes some people more sensitive to sunlight.) Another herb that may ease mild depression is *Ginkgo biloba*.

Counseling and therapy

Discussing your problems with a trained therapist can help when dealing with either anxiety or depression..

Cognitive therapy is one counseling approach. It encourages people to change their ways of thinking about themselves and the world. These beliefs often include convictions that bad experiences in the past are bound to be repeated in the future. Once the person discovers that this is not necessarily true and breaks the mental habit of thinking in such ways, he or she can take positive steps toward leading a more satisfying life.

There are other forms of therapy that can help with anxiety and depression. Among them are self-help groups, in which individuals discuss their feelings with each other, with or without a trained therapist present. Some people prefer this type of therapeutic setting to one-on-one counseling, or graduate to it after they engage in solo counseling.

If you feel that formal therapy will not suit you, then consider taking a creative approach to events that bother you. Writing or painting are good outlets for people who find it hard to reveal deep feelings, or who have nobody they can talk to.

Controlling your life is important in combating anxiety. You can do this by learning assertiveness techniques (see page 72), which can give you the confidence to change your circumstances. Exercise is another good approach. Researchers at the University of Massachusetts Center for Health and Fitness found that after subjects took a brisk 40-minute walk, their anxiety levels dropped.

CHAPTER 4

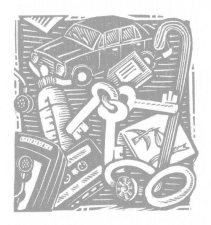

STRESS
AND THE
INDIVIDUAL

We all react to stress in our own ways.
An event that makes one person anxious will
be shrugged off by another, with barely a second
thought. Our response to stress is governed by a
number of different factors—age, health, intelligence.
However, the most dominant is our personality.
By learning how to assert ourselves, we can
offset the debilitating effects of stress.

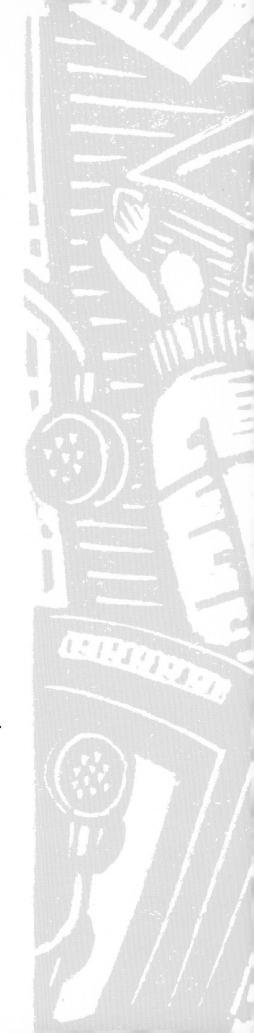

THE STAGES OF LIFE

Every age has its special challenges and unique stressors. At each stage new strategies for coping with stress need to be learned and previous ones modified, to live happily and healthfully.

Although the human lifespan has increased considerably since Shakespeare's day, the seven ages the Bard described remain much the same. However, the amount of time spent in each period and the problems encountered there differ.

CHILDHOOD

Children need extra help in developing skills for coping with problems, and adults are their best teachers. The problems may be minor, like frustration at physical incompetence, or more devastating, like the breakup of the family, but all will provoke a reaction. Any child who becomes aggressive, withdrawn, or "difficult" is under stress and in need of immediate attention. It is vital, therefore, that parents or teachers be alert to signs of pressure in children.

To ward off potential long-term problems, a responsible adult must react quickly and appropriately. For example, a mother

DEALING WITH COMMON PROBLEMS AT ALL STAGES OF LIFE

LIFE STAGE	GENERAL PROBLEMS	SPECIFIC STRESSES	COMMON REACTIONS	WHAT CAN BE DONE
CHILDHOOD				
	Physical mastery, competence, and coordination	Frustration: "I can't do it"	Tantrums	**By parents:**
		Difficulties with communication	Playing hooky and bullying	Be calm and supportive
	Intellectual mastery		Uncooperativeness	Communicate
		Jealousy toward brothers or sisters	Moodiness	Understand
	Emotional containment and maturity		Dependency	Be realistic about child's capabilities
		Adjusting to school	Bed-wetting	
		Rivalries with other school children and friends	Aggression	Set clear guidelines for behavior
			Withdrawal	
ADOLESCENCE				
	Acquiring independence and self-reliance	Anxieties about having friends, and over appearance (especially "being fat" for girls)	Eating disorders	**By parents:**
			Rudeness	As far as possible be supportive, positive, encouraging
	Establishment of peer group relations		Withdrawn behavior and secretiveness	
		Loneliness		Communicate parental anxieties
	Consolidation and development of earlier learning	Worries about schoolwork and getting into college	Refusal to keep "house rules"	**By child and parents:**
	Developing sexual identity	Conflicts about forming intimate relationships	Neglect of, or obsession with, schoolwork	For serious problems, seek family therapy
	Need for challenges and practice in skills to achieve competency	Exam pressure	Sexual adventurousness	Minimize power struggle by setting "house rules" together
		Pressure to achieve	Solvent abuse	

whose two-year-old child has become aggressive after the birth of a sibling should realize her toddler is fearful of losing parental attention. The mother can allay this fear by paying her toddler extra attention and setting aside special times for just the two of them to do things together. The parents of a schoolchild who seems withdrawn should try to discover what is making their child unhappy. Above all, they need to be supportive of their child. Having frank discussions with teachers will make it clear that they are concerned and would like to enlist their aid.

ADOLESCENCE

Once they reach their teens, young people must balance the need to develop apart from their families with the desire to retain their childhood security. Teens are pressured to conform with their peers, to perform well at school, and to meet the challenges of becoming competent in an adult world.

The adults in teenagers' lives need to be alert for signs of irritability, aggression, or withdrawal, and to make it clear that they are always available for them. A listening and nonjudgmental ear is an excellent antidote to stress, and this may be all your teenager needs to stay stress-free.

At difficult times, perhaps when a relationship goes bad, adolescents are best taught to deal with emotional upset by example. If you can express your own feelings and look after yourself when things get tough, your children will learn that the people who take care of themselves are the ones who cope best under pressure.

YOUTH

The major challenge of this period is to take full responsibility for finding one's own direction in the world. For an individual who does not know what he would like to do, schools often have guidance counseling, which may help. Counselors can pinpoint

DEALING WITH COMMON PROBLEMS AT ALL STAGES OF LIFE

GENERAL PROBLEMS	SPECIFIC STRESSES	COMMON REACTIONS	WHAT CAN BE DONE	LIFE STAGE
YOUTH				
Establishing independence at home or leaving to be on one's own Finding direction for education, training, or work Exploring possible long-term relationships	Conflict over leaving home Achieving financial independence Choice of college or other degree courses Worry about getting a job Concerns over finding "the right person"	Using home as a hotel Refusal to communicate or explain Being reckless with finances Sexual experimentation Overdependent relationships	**By parents:** Make clear limits of parental contribution Suggest career and financial advisers Listen without judging **By young adult:** Draw up budgets	
ADULTHOOD				
Establishment of permanent adult relationship, usually marriage Raising children Maintenance of financial viability Development of career	Finding a suitable spouse Career change Birth of children/infertility Worries about children Unemployment Moving to new locale Problems at work Separation and/or divorce	Burying oneself in work to avoid problems at home Drinking to forget Overindulging in spending or gambling Depression or illness, especially one which has a psychosomatic component—migraine or colitis Obesity	Honestly acknowledge problems Talk with spouse Join support group for specific problems Seek counseling for marital, financial, or career problems Turn to friends for peer-group support	

things that may be holding a student back, such as hidden fears or lack of confidence, and help to overcome these problems.

On the other hand, things may seem to be going very well, but because the pressure to maintain progress is great, youths may be prone to angry confrontations with friends or superiors; this, too, is a sign of stress. Engaging in physical activity can help release pent-up feelings.

ADULTHOOD

According to Freud, the essence of adult life is love and work, that is finding a loving partner and making the best contribution you can in your work life. These challenges are rarely completed without difficulty. While the average individual may be able to cope with the inevitable marital conflicts and problems of child-rearing, stress at work can compound the whole family's stress. Work overload can be alleviated by managing time better and setting priorities.

Nurturing relationships and honing parenting skills can make family life happier and more harmonious. There are many self-help books and adult education courses that aim to help people improve their interpersonal skills, but if relationships become very troubled, marriage or family counseling may become necessary (see also page 98).

MIDLIFE

This is the prime of life, a time when most people give to others the benefit of their experience. In other words, potentially it can be a satisfying period. Unfortunately, however, it may also be a time of the so-called midlife crisis, if one has not achieved all the dreams of youth and realizes that time is running out to do so.

When the latter is true, then it is important to find new meaning in life, but some people deny that anything has changed. For this reason, many marriages become strained or break up. A more positive approach is to

DEALING WITH COMMON PROBLEMS AT ALL STAGES OF LIFE

LIFE STAGE	GENERAL PROBLEMS	SPECIFIC STRESSES	COMMON REACTIONS	WHAT CAN BE DONE
MIDLIFE				
	Recognizing limitations of professional or career development	Lack of further promotion or possible unemployment	Depression	Review life and its possibilities
	Regret for chances or opportunities missed	Discontent with work, boredom, disillusionment	Irritability	Focus on positive aspects of life
	Recognition that procreative life and youth are probably over	Disagreements with children	Lack of motivation	Pay more attention to relationships—perhaps try a marriage-enrichment program
	Departure of children, signaling end of part of one's life	Dwindling physical powers and energy	Bitterness	Develop new interests and hobbies
	Denial of own mortality and ending of first half of life	Changes in physical appearance	Criticism of spouse, family, employer	Make changes to lifestyle
	Aging parents making demands on time and money	Forcing self to behave like a younger person	Attempts to preserve youth, often quite inappropriately—for example, dress, choice of partner, behavior	Make inancial plans to help eliminate future problems
	Older children marrying	Coping with aging parents' needs	Wanting to start anew	Initiate reretirement planning for next stage
		Changes in libido and sexual abilities	Resentment and jealousy of friends	Begin therapy, if necessary
		Development of health problems		Try relaxation techniques such as meditation
		Divorcing of deserting spouse		Take care of health—eat better, stop smoking, cut down on drinking, begin regular exercise

acknowledge changes and to see this period as a time of opportunity. Now is the time when many women, free of the concerns of child-rearing, go back to work on a full-time basis, while many men find themselves at a different crossroads. They can choose to continue with their careers, change course completely, or give work less priority in their lives and devote more time to their families and other interests.

During retirement, there is more time to spend on favorite pastimes, study, travel, or simply being with loved ones. Some retirees even start a second career or a part-time business. Research has shown that people who have a number of interests adapt best to retirement. Yoga, which can be taken up at any age, is beneficial in promoting sleep and general well-being at this stage of life. (See pages 56-57.)

RETIREMENT

The challenge in the years after 60 is to explore new possibilities in oneself while becoming reconciled to some changes in the status quo, for example, the loss of work and physical vigor; the death of friends and relatives; a drop in income; the winding down of one's social life; and anxiety over financial security. All of these concerns can result in depression, so planning ahead is vital. When these years are well planned, retirement can bring many joys.

OLD AGE

Now is the time to let go of many responsibilities and simply to enjoy the freedom to be with friends, children, grandchildren, and great grandchildren without having any time constraints. Consider joining a club that will provide companions and a range of social activities. While despondency can be a danger at this stage, especially if there is illness, the more active and independent you can be, the greater the chance that you will be able to live life to the fullest.

DEALING WITH COMMON PROBLEMS AT ALL STAGES OF LIFE

GENERAL PROBLEMS	SPECIFIC STRESS	COMMON REACTIONS	WHAT CAN BE DONE	LIFE STAGE
RETIREMENT				
Need to reconcile self to absence of a job and accompanying issues of social status Financial adjustment Prospect of illness or death	Loss of work-related social life Changing structure of the day Sense of loneliness and meaninglessness Anxieties about money, home, illness, aches, and pains	Depression Withdrawal Isolation Developing rigid routines: "I never go out at night" or "I always eat at 6:00 P.M." Inability to discuss problems with spouse/children Closer involvement with religious institution	Find new social context: join clubs or special-interest groups or move to retirement community. spend more time with family and younger people Become more involved in public sector—perhaps doing volunteer work in community	
OLD AGE				
Declining mental and physical powers Possible financial anxieties Loss of independence	Forgetfulness Illness Weakness and dependence Loss of home Death of friends and family members	Depression Lack of interest in life Personal neglect Bitterness Anger Fear and mistrust Becoming secretive	Choose best possible physical care—modified house or apartment, sharing home of child, private nurses, or nursing home Maintain interest in family circle or other social outlets	

DAY-TO-DAY STRESS

No one is immune from everyday stress. New demands in life, even pleasant ones, can make stress levels intolerable. Here are ways to monitor and modify stress before it gets out of hand.

The fact that major stressful events can affect a person's physical and mental well-being has been well known for some time. But not until recently has it been recognized that the cumulative effect of a number of small stresses can cause the same amount of damage.

In the early 1970's, Thomas Holmes and Richard Rahe, working at the University of Washington, looked at the effect a series of expected events can have on a person's life. They found that any change—even a positive one—can cause stress. To measure the degree of stress that a person had suffered

PERSONAL STRESSFUL EVENT SCALE

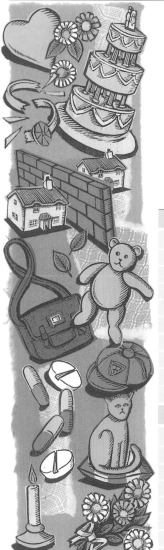

Not everyone is affected by events in the same way. Even when life is stressful, some people cope better than others. If you have experienced what you consider a great deal of stress within a short time, your health could be at risk.

The following chart, developed by Cary L. Cooper, Rachel D. Cooper, and Lynn H. Eaker in their book *Living with Stress,* was designed to measure your stress levels. First

look at the chart and see if any of the events match your experience in the past two years. Then, on a separate piece of paper, jot down the number that best expresses the degree of stress that the event caused you (1 indicates minimal stress and 10 maximum stress). Add up your score. Fifty points is an average stress level. A higher score indicates recurring problems that may prove to be too heavy a burden.

RELATIONSHIPS	1	2	3	4	5	6	7	8	9	10
Engagement										
Marriage										
Arguments with partner										
Marital problems										
Problem relatives										
Problem friends										
Problem neighbors										
End of long-term relationship										
Separation from loved one										
Divorce										
PARENT/CHILD										
Pregnancy										
Childbirth										
Birth of grandchildren										
Disagreements with children										
Disagreements with parents										
Child starts school										
Child leaves home										
Child marries										

over a period of time, they created an index that listed 43 of the most common stressful episodes in an average individual's life and rated each one for stressfulness. Death of a spouse had the highest rating, 100, and minor violations of the law the lowest, 11. The researchers found that subjects with a score of over 150 had a 31 percent chance of developing a health problem within two years; subjects who scored over 300 stood a 79 percent chance of illness, unless effective measures were taken to combat stress. Although Holmes and Rahe's work demonstrated that a relationship exists between stress and illness, it did not take into account individual differences in reacting to stress. So current thinking is that the most important factor in assessing stress is how individuals rate its effects.

Pathway to health

If you are constantly under a great deal of stress, developing habits that help you relax every day is a good way to cope. Try one or more of the following: meditation (page 42), tai chi (page 36), progressive relaxation (page 39), yoga (page 56), an aromatherapy bath (page 68), or a brisk walk of at least 20 minutes.

Laughter is also good for relieving stress, so take home an amusing video to watch, or tune into a favorite comedy show. A change in lifestyle can be beneficial, too. Cut down on smoking and overeating, and drink alcoholic and caffeinated beverages in moderation.

PERSONAL STRESSFUL EVENT SCALE

ILLNESS/BEREAVEMENT	1	2	3	4	5	6	7	8	9	10
Illness of self										
Illness of family member										
Illness of relative										
Having to care for ill person										
Death of partner										
Death of child										
Death of relative										
Death of close friend										
EMPLOYMENT										
Work problems										
Promotion										
Demotion										
Job change										
Threatened loss of work										
Unemployment										
Retirement										
FINANCE/GENERAL										
Home improvements										
House purchase										
Moving house										
Sale of home										
Building work										
Increased borrowings										
Debt problem										
Insurance problem										
Legal problem										
TOTALS										
GRAND TOTAL										

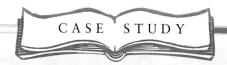

A Woman of a Certain Age

Middle age can be a stressful time for many women. They may have anxieties about grown children starting out in the world and worries over aging parents, plus the first signs of the menopause. When additional problems arise—for example, unemployment or debt—stress levels can reach the point where health is seriously affected.

Sally, a devoted wife and mother, is just about to turn 50. There are a number of disquieting changes going on in her life. Jenny, her 18-year-old daughter, is going away to college in the fall, and the prospect of her only child leaving home is upsetting. Tuition is high and Sally is worried that she and her husband Joe might not be able to carry the full cost, especially since they have very little money set aside for their own retirement. Sally is anxious about looking for work. Before her marriage to Joe 25 years ago, she was a kindergarten teacher, but she has not worked since.

Adding to her concerns is the failing health of her father. For the past few months, he has become increasingly more frail and she is worried that he will have to hire a nurse, move in with her and Joe, or move to a nursing home. On top of all this, Sally has become aware of changes to her mood and body. She has had a number of hot flashes and unexplained mood swings and wonders if she may be starting the menopause.

Given these pressures, it is no wonder that Sally is feeling tense and irritable. She has trouble sleeping at night, has lost all interest in sex, and suffers from continual low-grade aches and pains. She cannot remember the last time she felt so completely besieged by worries and unable to cope with them.

CHILDREN
While children's growing independence is gratifying, the idea of their leaving home—creating an empty nest—can be very distressing.

FINANCES
Family purses can be strained by dependent older children, elderly parents, health problems, or the need to put away money for retirement.

HUSBAND
In midlife themselves, husbands may be facing flagging physical capacities and the stresses of early retirement or possible unemployment.

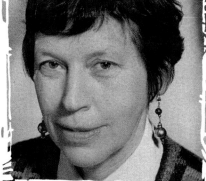

PARENTS
Becoming increasingly infirm, elderly parents often are dependent on their middle-aged children. Some need financial assistance; others need help with everyday chores.

WORK
The prospect of returning to work full time after a long absence can cause great anxiety.

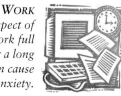

PERSONAL HEALTH
Midlife is the time of the menopause. Changes in hormonal production may cause depression, inability to concentrate, and a host of physical symptoms.

WHAT SALLY SHOULD DO

Stress is greatest when a person feels overwhelmed and powerless. Thus Sally needs to attack each of her problems separately. The first problem to address is her own health. Much of Sally's depression and physical symptoms could be related to menopausal changes; she should see a gynecologist.

Sally needs to confront her feelings about Jenny leaving home. Rather than anticipating loneliness, she could look upon this time as a new start for herself. Sally might want to consider getting a job, especially since money is a major concern. Returning to the workforce after a long absence can be unsettling, but she could start gradually, doing volunteer work a day or two at the local elementary school.

Whether Sally's father goes into a nursing home or moves in with her is dependent on a number of factors. She and her husband must talk about what they can and cannot afford, as well as how such a move would impact on their marriage and family life. They need to be as realistic as possible, especially if Sally is planning to find a full-time job.

They might want to see a certified financial planner who would be able to provide them with a budget plan that would take into consideration their need to save for retirement, the extra costs of having a child in college, as well as caring for an elderly parent.

Action Plan

CHILDREN
Accept that Jenny has to begin to live an independent life. Ask her if she could work part time to defray school costs and if she has fully investigated all possible scholarship opportunities.

PARENTS
Arrange to speak to a financial consultant and a geriatric specialist, together with her father. Discuss the possibility of giving Sally power of attorney.

FINANCES
Scout around for good financial advice. Discuss with a financial adviser the best way of budgeting their finances. Consider getting a full- or part-time job.

HUSBAND
Stress typically spills over into one's relationship. Be sure to spend some time together alone. Arrange a "date" for every Friday night—be it dinner out or staying in and watching a movie.

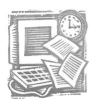

HEALTH
Make an appointment with a gynecologist. Read up on treatments to relieve menopausal distress. Try some self-help relaxation techniques that can be done at home. Start walking a half hour each day.

WORK
Contact local schools to see if substitute teachers are needed. Consider taking courses that would bring her teaching certificate up-to-date. Visit an employment agency to discuss her prospects in other areas.

HOW THINGS TURNED OUT FOR SALLY

Sally's gynecologist confirmed her menopausal status and prescribed estrogen replacement therapy (ERT). Within a few weeks her hot flashes had ceased and her depression abated. She felt more cheerful and energetic and able to tackle the new challenges in her life.

Unfortunately, her father's health deteriorated rapidly. After talking it over, they moved him into their home as soon as Jenny left, and Sally arranged for a nurse to come in part time every day to help him

The sale of her father's apartment eased Sally's financial worries for the time being, but she thought she should start looking into retirement plans and also find a job. Although she was very nervous about returning to work after 25 years, she found that she was excit-ed about the prospect. After some research, she discovered that there were a number of openings for day-care teachers. She obtained a job working at a nearby day-care center three days a week.

Jenny was doing well in college. In the summer, she found a job working with her mother, and she enjoyed it so much she decided to major in early child education.

Aromatherapy

For hundreds of years, people have used the essential oils that give various plants their scents to relax the body and mind. These treatments, known as aromatherapy, are increasingly being used to combat disorders and work-induced stress.

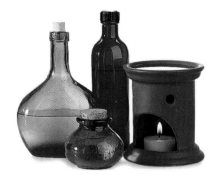

VERSATILE OILS
Essential oils are contained in certain bath and massage oils. You can vaporize them over an incense burner if they are first added to water.

Aromatherapy heals through our sense of smell, the most well developed of the five senses, and by absorption of a plant's essence through the skin. Certain scents can invigorate or induce calm. Particular essences can speed the soothing of an aching back and tense muscles during an aromatherapy massage.

Aromatherapists divide the oils into three groups. Uplifting oils, for example, bergamot, basil, and rosemary, invigorate the body and raise the spirits. Calming oils such as cedarwood, jasmine, and neroli have a sedating effect. Toning and regulating oils, such as lemongrass, and myrrh (not to be used during

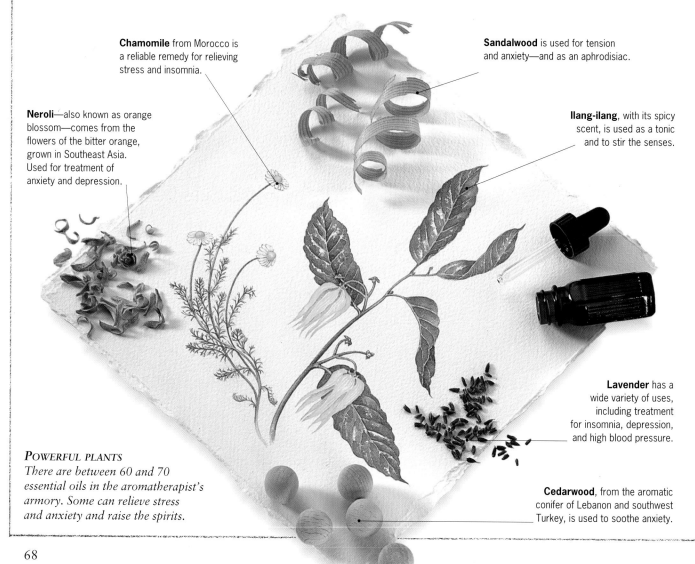

Chamomile from Morocco is a reliable remedy for relieving stress and insomnia.

Neroli—also known as orange blossom—comes from the flowers of the bitter orange, grown in Southeast Asia. Used for treatment of anxiety and depression.

Sandalwood is used for tension and anxiety—and as an aphrodisiac.

Ilang-ilang, with its spicy scent, is used as a tonic and to stir the senses.

Lavender has a wide variety of uses, including treatment for insomnia, depression, and high blood pressure.

POWERFUL PLANTS
There are between 60 and 70 essential oils in the aromatherapist's armory. Some can relieve stress and anxiety and raise the spirits.

Cedarwood, from the aromatic conifer of Lebanon and southwest Turkey, is used to soothe anxiety.

pregnancy) are said to condition the skin and promote the health of the internal organs. Vaporizing such essential oils as jasmine or lavender over a burner can bring a calming atmosphere to your home or office. You may unwind after a hard day at work by giving yourself a shoulder and neck massage using the oils of rose, sandalwood, or chamomile.

Oils are also relaxing in baths, in face packs and foot soaks, or as an inhalation (see below). Essential oils can be bought at health food and body-care shops. They should be stored in a cool place (but not in a refrigerator) and kept out of the reach of children.

Most oils are extracted by distillation. Depending on the plant, the seeds, flowers, leaves, bark, or resin are placed in a container and steam is passed through them. The oils first evaporate, then condense when the steam cools; after this process they can be separated out from the water. Very large quantities are needed— for instance, it can take about 4,400 pounds of rose petals to make just 1 quart of rose oil. For this reason, the oils are quite expensive, but only a few drops are used at one time.

> ## WARNING
> If you are, or might be, pregnant, seek advice from a qualified aromatherapist or your doctor before using essential oils; some oils can harm your unborn baby.
>
> If you have allergies, a medical problem, or have recently been ill or involved in an accident, consult your physician to find out if you should use aromatherapy, including massage.

USING THE OILS

Never apply undiluted oils directly to your skin; they should always be mixed with a suitable medium— warm water or a light, mild base oil. If you have sensitive skin, apply only a drop or two of the diluted oil at first, and wait to see the results.

Everyone has favorite aromas, so try out a range of oils to discover which you like best, as well as which ones are the most effective for each purpose.

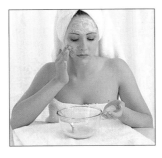

FACE PACK
Mix 1 teaspoon of cold-pressed wheat germ or almond oil with 1 drop of essential oil. Rose suits most skin types; tea tree is good for oily skin. Stir in 3 teaspoons of live, whole-milk yogurt and $\frac{1}{2}$ to 1 teaspoon of fine oatmeal to form a paste. Apply a thin layer of the mixture to your face and leave for 10 to 15 minutes. Rinse off with cool water.

BATH
Ensure that the bathroom is warm and all windows shut so that the vapors will not escape. Add 6 to 10 drops of oil to hot bathwater and swish this around so that an oily film forms on the surface. When you get in, some of the oil will penetrate your skin, and you will inhale more through the steam.

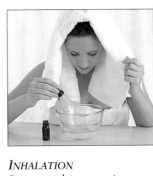

INHALATION
Pour very hot water into a bowl and add 2 to 3 drops of cedarwood or juniper essential oil. Position your face above the rising steam, then cover your head and the bowl with a towel and inhale and exhale deeply until the water cools.

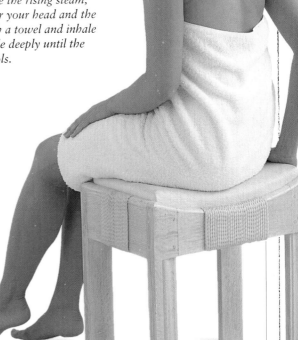

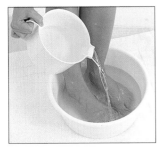

FOOT SOAK
Fill a small tub or large bowl half full with hot water. Add up to 10 drops of rosemary, peppermint, or lavender essential oil. Soak your feet for 10 minutes and dry them well. Then massage gently.

TACKLING THE STRESS IN YOUR LIFE

Not having control over important facets of your life is stressful. No matter what your personality, you can use assertiveness to gain back control and cut down on stress.

THE TORTOISE AND THE HARE
Characteristics of people of Types A and B are described in Aesop's well-known fable with the hare being Type A and the tortoise Type B.

No two human beings are alike. Almost from the moment of birth, a baby asserts an individual personality and temperament. As life goes on, these characteristics are further shaped by each person's experiences.

Even though most of us acknowledge that everyone is different, we still try to group people according to types. For thousands of years, philosophers, theologians, and scientists the world over have devised various systems that classify people by their physique, intelligence, or emotions, in an effort to understand how and why they behave the way they do. A number of modern psychologists have created psychological classifications to describe different personality types, in order to better treat emotional and personality disorders.

BODY TYPES

In the 1940's, W. H. Sheldon of Harvard University developed Kretchmer's concept of somatotypes. This characterizes people according to three distinctive physical shapes, each of which has a distinct personality. An endomorph has an overall rounded shape and head with a heavy build and a predisposition for storing fat. An endomorph's personality is supposedly relaxed and easy-going like this shape.

The ectomorph is sharp and thin in form, with spindly legs and arms, and not much muscle or fat. Matching their physical forms, ectomorphs are said to be tense, taut, sensitive, introverted, and artistic.

A mesomorph has an athletic form, with a lot of muscle but not much fat, a large head, broad shoulders, and relatively narrow hips. The mesomorph is said to be energetic, aggressive, and competitive.

While the somatotype theory was largely discredited in later decades, health-care professionals still acknowledge that some body shapes do have health implications.

The apple-shaped individual, with large deposits of fat located on the abdomen, is much more prone to heart disease and breast cancer than are pear-shaped or bean-pole shaped people. Control of weight through diet and exercise can help to reduce these risks for many persons.

PERSONALITY TYPES

In the early 1900's, Sigmund Freud, an Austrian neurologist and founder of psychoanalysis, divided personality into three parts: the id (representing our instinctive and unconscious wants and needs), the superego (standing for the often admonishing voice of society), and the ego (our conscious "I," which tries to reconcile the conflicts between the id and superego).

Freud's groundbreaking work provided a springboard for his famous student, Carl Jung, a Swiss psychologist. Jung classified people into two major groups—introverts and extroverts—according to their social and emotional interaction. Introverts are restrained, retiring individuals, often shy and unforthcoming around others, but who maintain reserves of thoughtfulness, independence, and quiet determination. Their opposites, extroverts, are characterized as energetic and outgoing, at ease in company, and adaptable and flexible team members. Confident and outspoken with others, they require the stimulation other people can give to perform well, and are therefore often less at ease with solitude.

While classifying people by personality type was considered important in treating mental health problems, it was not often used to determine physical ailments. This changed in the early 1960's with the pioneering work of two American cardiologists, Meyer Friedman and Ray Rosenman. While treating people with heart disease, they were puzzled by the fact that more than half of their heart attack patients did not have the usual risk factors of high cholesterol, hypertension, obesity, or cigarette smoking. What was causing their heart disease? Careful observation revealed that these patients had similar personalities. They were all competitive, ambitious, and driven by deadlines. Friedman and Rosenman called this aggressive personality trait Type A and developed a test to determine which people had Type A personalities. The Type A individuals were constantly involved

TABLE OF THE HUMORS

The ancient Greek physicians, Hippocrates and Galen, and the Elizabethans in England, believed that there were four personality types—sanguine or happy, melancholic or sad, choleric or angry, and phlegmatic or listless. Each personality type was thought to be the result of an excess of a particular humor or body fluid—blood, black bile, yellow bile, or phlegm. The humors were related to the four elements—fire or blood, earth or black bile, air or yellow bile, and water or phlegm.

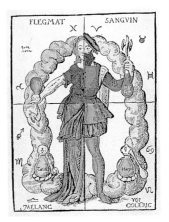

ELEMENTAL TYPES
Elizabethans believed everyone had a surfeit of one humor.

PERSONALITY AND YOUR HEALTH

According to some philosophies, certain character traits and physical features have the potential to affect one's health. You can check the chart to see how you may be at risk, but keep in mind that these are abbreviated and broadly stroked descriptions. Most people have a mixture of elements and do not fit one category precisely.

CATEGORIZATION	PERSONALITY AND CHARACTER TRAITS	HEALTH FACTORS
ANCIENT INDIAN PHILOSOPHY		
Hindu philosophers believed that the life energy (*prana*) is manifested in the human body according to the five elements—ether, air, fire, water, and earth in their three basic compound forms—*vata* (air and ether), *pitta* (fire and water) and *kapha* (water and earth).	**Vata:** Small-boned, wiry people, often nervous types, unable to sit still for long. At times highly intelligent, but often abstract rather than practical, and lacking humor.	Susceptible to constipation, arthritis, lower back problems, and lung disorders.
	Pitta: Intense, hardworking people, often with athletic, muscular bodies. Highly energetic with curiosity and a hunger for learning, and prone to impatience and jealousy.	Prone to cancers, strokes, and digestive, blood, and hormone deficiency disorders.
	Kapha: Often stocky and thick-set people with a tendency to put on weight easily. Slow moving, solid, jolly, and emotionally stable, they like the status quo, enjoy the good things in life, and are perhaps a little unimaginative.	A tendency to succumb to illnesses affecting the lungs, lymph glands, and stomach. A sluggish circulation may affect the heart.
TYPES A AND B		
Psychologists use these convenient tags to describe a person's attitudes toward time and tasks, self-image, and self-evaluation.	**Type A:** A self-centered personality, incessantly driven to achieve more and more in less and less time, in competition with other things and other people. Always running "at full throttle," ambitious and insecure.	Type A's are more likely to suffer infections and are 80 percent more prone to hypertension and cardiovascular disease than B's.
	Type B: People lacking in Type A traits. Unhurried, relaxed, patient, and quietly self-assured, with little need to prove themselves. They pace themselves and their work well, but perhaps they are a little lacking in drive.	Type B's are not as susceptible to heart disease, but have a higher incidence of depression than Type A's.
CHINESE PHILOSOPHY		
In traditional Chinese thought, personality is made up of two opposing attractions—*yin* and *yang*, the female and male forces in nature. Their mutual attraction is the source of all movement and energy—the life force called *chi*.	**Yins:** "Dark and moist" yins are tranquil, quietly reflective types, mentally alert but also passive personalities who make better followers than leaders.	An excess of yin can lead to sluggishness and deficiencies of some sort, such as underactive organs and pale complexions.
	Yangs: "Bright, hot, and dry" characters, who are active strivers, are physically more than mentally active, and good leader material, but who are also aggressive, undisciplined, and uncooperative with others.	An excess of yang produces symptoms associated with heat, such as fever, sweating, and flushes.

CALM YOURSELF

Should you become angry, try the following tactics to defuse your emotions.

▶ *Count to 10.*

▶ *Speak slowly and deliberately.*

▶ *Lower your voice.*

▶ *Cross your fingers and breathe deeply and slowly.*

▶ *Go for a short walk.*

in many different activities and felt a driving need to compete and win. They had a marked tendency toward aggressive and hostile feelings. They appeared to be unable to relax —hurrying their lives away by eating, walking, and talking very quickly. In short, they were in a constant state of mental and physical hypervigilance. Those who did not share these character traits were called Type B's. Type B's were the opposite of Type A's, in that they were more relaxed and easygoing.

Using their personality test, Friedman and Rosenman were amazed to find that Type A's had twice the rate of heart attacks and heart disease than Type B's. For the first time, personality was being used to determine physical health. But the question remained: what was causing heart disease in the Type A patients? Friedman and Rosenman concluded that the hard-driving personality and overly demanding behavior of Type A patients were causing their heart problems. The treatment seemed obvious: help Type A people to modify their behavior so that they could deal with stress more effectively. In short, teach them to become more like Type B's.

Later research, however, showed that not all Type A's had heart attacks and that not

all Type B's were free of heart disease. Researchers reconsidered the relevance of determining the risk of heart disease according to the degree of free-floating anger and hostility people felt. They found a definite correlation between anger and blocked coronary arteries. Subsequent research has shown that anger and hostility literally take a toll on the heart.

MANAGING ANGER

Anger, linked with hostility, puts a person on the alert, and triggers the fight-or-flight response with all its attendant physiological responses. Some people believe that if they vent their anger, they will not experience any ill effects, physically or psychologically. They might express it directly by shouting at the person who caused it, or indirectly, perhaps by hitting a pillow. Neither of these strategies, however, is effective at stopping the effects of anger. Suppressing anger does not work either.

The best way to deal with anger is try to avoid it in the first place. This may mean giving in sometimes, or sidestepping conflict. But better yet is to make your feelings known before you reach the boiling point. For example, if your children annoy you by tracking mud into the house, simply cleaning up after them will not solve the problem—eventually you will explode in a torrent of angry words. The best solution is to express your feelings about muddy floors in a calm, straightforward way and to tell your children that you expect them to wipe their feet before entering the house. The technique used for doing this is known as assertion (see page 74), and it is one of the key strategies for reducing stress levels. By solving a problem before it becomes a crisis, you will find that you feel less tense and are able to cope better with small annoyances.

ASSERTING YOURSELF

The foundation of assertion is that every person has rights. Being assertive means being confident that you have the right to express your feelings. It also means that you remain aware of another person's rights. In this way, you can avoid conflict because you are not attempting to say that your rights and needs are more important than another's. By taking the rights of others seriously, you ensure that the other person takes your rights seriously, too. Also, by

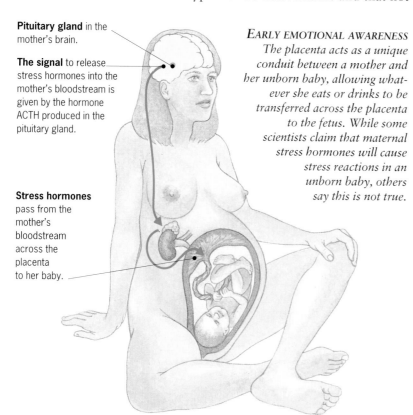

Pituitary gland in the mother's brain.

The signal to release stress hormones into the mother's bloodstream is given by the hormone ACTH produced in the pituitary gland.

Stress hormones pass from the mother's bloodstream across the placenta to her baby.

EARLY EMOTIONAL AWARENESS The placenta acts as a unique conduit between a mother and her unborn baby, allowing whatever she eats or drinks to be transferred across the placenta to the fetus. While some scientists claim that maternal stress hormones will cause stress reactions in an unborn baby, others say this is not true.

becoming more assertive, you will find that you can tell people how you feel. You will be able to say no when you want to, and refuse unreasonable demands.

Why be assertive?

While being assertive is a sensible approach, acting assertively can be difficult. Many people prefer to avoid conflict and give in without a fight. They often apologize repeatedly for small infractions and begin far too many sentences with "I'm sorry." These old habits can be hard to break.

If you feel you are not assertive enough, take some time to think about the areas in your life where assertion would help. Do you wish you could tell people at work what you want? Or that you could make it known to your spouse that you want help with the housework? Do you feel that your friends never ask you what you want to do when you go out together? Or that you never seem able to ask your physician to explain things more clearly? Make a list of the situations in which you would like to be more assertive.

Community colleges, continuing education programs, and the like offer classes in assertiveness training that teach simple techniques. These will enable you to change from a passive person to someone who knows how to make sure your needs are addressed. The secret of true assertiveness is to identify and understand passivity and aggression, and to recognize that passive reactions, such as withdrawal, sulkiness, or reproach, are not only inadequate but also ineffective as a rule.

The language of assertion

The first step in asserting yourself is to be clear about what you want. The next step is to make the other person aware of it by saying it simply, clearly, and directly. Before you speak, take a moment or two to collect your thoughts. For instance if someone has overcharged you, say, "You've given me the wrong change. I think you'll find that I gave you $10, not $5." Try to be direct and to the point, avoiding a long explanation. Speak firmly, but be polite. If the person you are talking to is not helpful, you may need to repeat your request, or make a further suggestion: "If you look in the cash register, I think you'll find that I gave you a $10 bill." Continue to repeat

ASSERTIVE BEHAVIOR
Simple, straightforward steps can help to resolve problems.

Identify the problem

Approach the person

Explain the benefits

Explain the consequences

Problem resolved

Be patient

Maintain communication

your request, remaining calm and polite. If the person refuses to acknowledge your complaint and check the register, then summarize the situation as it stands and state that you will seek out the next level of authority. For example, you could say, "I see you will not check the register. I would like to speak with the store manager."

Practicing assertion techniques

You can practice being assertive on your own, by mentally rehearsing conversations. For example, you might plan a talk to your boss about something that has been troubling you at work. People respond best if you use the word "I," so that the emphasis is on what you want, rather than on what they have done wrong. Instead of saying "You always make me work through lunch and I am sick of it," try, "I value my lunch hour and would appreciate it if we could schedule the day's work so that I can take my lunch hour every day." This statement lets your employer know how you feel, but avoids apportioning blame. By using the word "we" and making a suggestion about how to solve the problem, you show that you want to be part of the solution.

When to compromise

Even the best assertiveness techniques in the world, however, do not always work. Sometimes it is necessary to give in. Some situations are difficult to resolve, either because they have been going on for a long

ASSERTION CHECKLIST

Not only what you say but but also your physical demeanor is important when trying to get across your point of view, make your feelings known, or ensure that your position is clear.

▶ *Stand up straight.*

▶ *Concentrate on breathing regularly to help keep your voice firm and even.*

▶ *Make eye contact; averting your eyes makes you look submissive and unsure of yourself. However, there's no need to stare either.*

▶ *Speak in a firm voice; do not shout or raise your voice.*

▶ *Stick to the point; avoid long explanations.*

▶ *Be polite but do not start a sentence with "I'm sorry."*

▶ *Listen to the other person's point of view but be persistent.*

continued on page 76

Using Assertion

Some people are happy speaking up whereas others find it very difficult to make their voices (and wishes) heard. By learning a few, easily mastered lessons in assertiveness, you will be able to get more from life.

AN INDIVIDUAL'S RIGHTS

You may feel better about what you want and who you are by thinking about some inalienable rights. These include:

▶ *The right to make mistakes.*

▶ *The right to refuse requests without feeling guilty.*

▶ *The right to express feelings.*

▶ *The right for your own needs to be considered as important as those of other people.*

▶ *The right to object to unfair criticism.*

Many of the problems individuals face are linked to their inability to take charge of their relationships at home or in the outside world. Nonassertive people allow their children and spouses free time, while they do all the chores, then sulk or explode in a rage in response to a small demand. At work they find themselves taking on tasks that are not their responsibility, working long hours, forgoing vacations, and then becoming ill. Nonassertive people do themselves no good. If they were more emphatic about their needs and feelings, everyone would gain. Children would learn self-reliance. Communication between spouses would likely improve. And companies would function better if their employees were not taking sick leave due to overwork and understaffing.

ASKING FOR A RAISE IN SALARY

When you ask for a raise, you should remember that you are entitled to have your worth recognized in a monetary form, just as your employer is free to grant or refuse your request. If your request is reasonable, your chances of success are good. But even if your request is well founded, you may be turned down because of extenuating circumstances. It is important to learn what these are, as rejection can play havoc with your self-esteem, not to mention your ability to assert yourself in other areas of your life.

Before you make an appointment with your employer, write down a complete list of the assets you bring to your work. You don't need to recite them all, but they will help you make it clear that you deserve more money, and the list itself will increase your confidence so that you will find it easier to be assertive when you do meet with your employer.

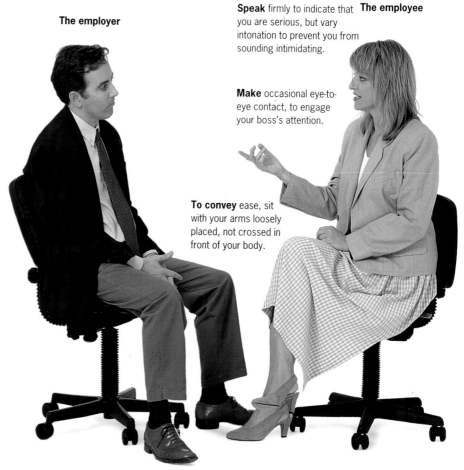

The employer

Speak firmly to indicate that you are serious, but vary intonation to prevent you from sounding intimidating. **The employee**

Make occasional eye-to-eye contact, to engage your boss's attention.

To convey ease, sit with your arms loosely placed, not crossed in front of your body.

HOW TO BE AN ASSERTIVE PERSON

An assertive person is "open and flexible, genuinely concerned with the rights of others, yet at the same time able to establish very well his or her own rights," according to a definition given by Alberti and Emmons in *Your Perfect Right: A Guide to Assertive Behavior.*

To achieve this ideal, you need first to identify the areas where you feel least confident. It could be at work or social gatherings, where people talk to you but you do not feel you have anything worthwhile to say; or it might be at home, where other people's needs take precedence over your own. Ask yourself what it is you want. Be specific, whether it's having someone else order office supplies or reminding your partner to buy milk on the way home from work. Next, repeat to yourself "An Individual's Rights" (see opposite page) until they are ingrained.

MAKING A COMPLAINT AT A STORE

An important assertiveness technique is to be persistent. We often lose in a conflict because we give up easily. The trick is to keep politely repeating what it is we want.

(see opposite page)

PASSIVE OR AGGRESSIVE?

Changing the way you speak can make you more assertive. Be direct and clear. "Please wash the dishes," is more to the point than "Am I the only one who cares that the kitchen is a mess?" When you want to be assertive, use assertive words. These include "I" statements such as "I think," "I feel," "I want." If you wish to be more co-operative, use "let's," or "we could." Remember, there are fundamental differences between assertiveness and aggression. When you are nonassertive you are denying your own rights, when aggressive, you are denying the rights of others.

The salesperson

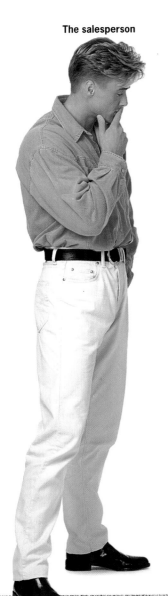

The shopper

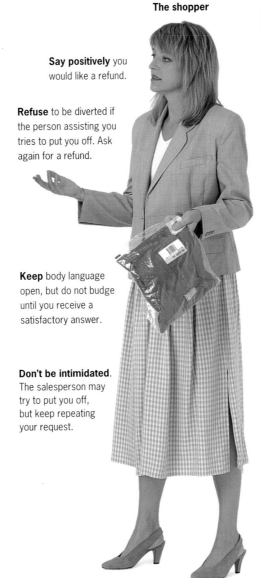

Say positively you would like a refund.

Refuse to be diverted if the person assisting you tries to put you off. Ask again for a refund.

Keep body language open, but do not budge until you receive a satisfactory answer.

Don't be intimidated. The salesperson may try to put you off, but keep repeating your request.

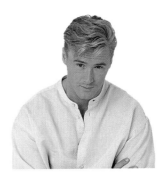

THE NONASSERTIVE RESPONSE
"That's okay, I don't mind. I will drop what I am doing and do it right now. No, no, I'm not busy."

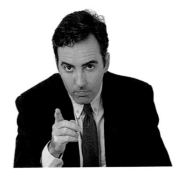

THE AGGRESSIVE RESPONSE
"What do you take me for? Why should I jump whenever you call? Find someone else to run around for you, I'm busy."

time or because the person you are negotiating with is in a stronger position.

For more challenging situations, it may help to practice what you want to say with a friend. Often, people who are learning to be assertive are afraid that they are being rude or aggressive. You could try role-playing with your friend taking the part of your adversary. Record or have someone videotape the session, to find out what you look and sound like. With this feedback you can then adjust your voice and manner, so that you are less aggressive or more assertive, as you deem necessary.

The bonuses of assertion

Acting assertively will not change your life overnight, but with practice and persistence, you should find that other people will respect you and your wishes more often. Instead of simmering inside with unresolved anger, you will be able to express your feelings and work with others to find a solution that respects the needs and wishes of all, without unnecessary confrontation. Being assertive will help you to be more self-confident and in control of your life, as you take active steps toward achieving what you really want.

ARE YOU ASSERTIVE?

Each one of us likes to have his or her point of view appreciated and considered. But humans are sociable beings, and expressing an opinion in the face of possible opposition does not always come easily.

How good are you at striking a balance between submissiveness and aggression? Add up your "yes" answers to the questions that are given below and compare your total with the results.

QUESTIONS	YES	NO
Do you avoid conflict with others at any cost, rather than argue with them, even over issues that are important to you?		
Do you feel that things seem to matter more to others than they do to you, and therefore make allowances for them, for the sake of peace?		
If a salesman, market researcher, or political canvasser calls you, do you find it difficult to tell him or her politely that you are not interested and then hang up?		
If something you purchased was faulty, would you keep it, but resolve to shop elsewhere in the future, rather than taking it back for repair or a refund?		
If someone pushes in front of you in the line, do you keep quiet and sulk, hoping the message will be clear rather than voicing your irritation?		
Are others' feelings always more important to you than the principle of the matter?		
When there's a deadline to meet at the office, are you always the one who stays late to finish it— even when you would rather not?		
Do you prefer your partner to make the shopping decisions?		
Do you drive or walk around for ages before stopping someone to ask for directions?		
Do you find yourself unable to say no to requests for a favor, and worry that you might be asked to do things you would rather not?		
Do you shy away from asking for advice because you are afraid of appearing incompetent?		
If you feel wounded by an unfair remark, do you add it to the stockpile of injuries, rather than firmly but politely correcting whoever said it?		
Do you feel embarrassed or overdemanding in telling your spouse what you want in your relationship?		
If someone makes a mistake, do you prefer to avoid mentioning it, rather than draw attention to it?		

HOW DID YOU SCORE ?

0 to 5 "yes" answers
Your score indicates that you could be a little more sympathetic to others. You seem to express your opinions more aggressively than is necessary or, indeed, warranted.

5 to 10 "yes" answers
You seem to have a reasonable approach to confrontation, and are able to balance your opinions with those of other people so that both of you are satisfied.

Over 10 "yes" answers
You appear to set a very low value on your rights and points of view. You are as important as anyone else, so be more decisive and express what you want.

CHAPTER 5

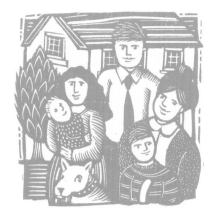

STRESS AND THE FAMILY

Because families consist of individuals with different personalities, desires, and needs that are changing all the time, conflict and stress are inevitable. By developing awareness of everyone's requirements and trying to balance them with plenty of give and take, stress within the family can be reduced. This chapter looks at some of the ways you can make your family life more relaxed and harmonious.

THE FAMILY UNIT

Today's families take many forms other than the traditional unit in which the father goes out to work and the mother stays home with the children. Each type has its own joys and stresses.

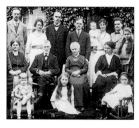

FAMILY TIES
Years ago, the extended family often spanned four generations. Now the family extends "horizontally" as well due to remarriage, resulting in stepchildren, new births, and the addition of the new spouse's family.

In many traditional cultures, people live with their parents until they marry, and afterward continue to live nearby. Each member of the extended family—parents, grandparents, children, aunts, uncles, and cousins—relies on the others for support, and several generations may live together in the same house. This sort of close family network has much in its favor: it can provide emotional balance, financial stability, a feeling of rootedness, and day-to-day support with child care and housework. It might not, however, allow young people a great deal of individual freedom and can give the older generations unwarranted license to interfere.

THE CHANGING FAMILY
In the West, the traditional extended family has been eroded by two major factors. The first is that in today's labor market people are relocating far more frequently to take up new jobs, and the second is a preference for smaller nuclear families, comprising only parents and a few children. But there are other factors as well. Since the 1960's the number of marital separations and divorces has escalated and the trend has grown for serial remarriage—marriage for a second or third time. There has also been a large increase in children born out of wedlock, so that more and more families are now headed by one parent only. These single parents are primarily women.

While some single parents return to their own parental homes with their children, in a re-creation of the extended family, others bring up their children alone. Sometimes divorced husbands and wives form binuclear families, where children divide their time between two households. Family life can be further complicated when one or both members of the divorced couple remarry and bring a stepfather or stepmother into their children's lives, possibly accompanied by stepbrothers and sisters.

THE STATE OF MARRIAGE

Recent statistics show that for every two marriages one ends in divorce, and the majority of divorcees remarry. The trend is slightly higher in the U.S., where there are more marriages and, proportionally, more divorces and remarriages.

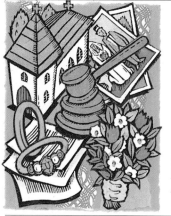

UNITED STATES (255,200,000)*	UNITED KINGDOM (57,700,000)*	GERMANY (80,300,000)*
MARRIAGE		
2,362,000	364,600	405,200
DIVORCE		
1,215,000	175,100	135,000
REMARRIAGE		
1,075,000	156,000	156,000

* These figures refer to the overall population of each country. The remaining figures are for 1992, except US remarriage, which has been estimated from 1988 figures.

The fluid nature of the modern family has made it all too easy to lose touch with members of an extended family. In addition, new people often have to be integrated into the larger family unit. It can be a challenge, with these conditions, to maintain a feeling of closeness with all your relatives. But frequently the desire to renew contact with them gets stronger as you grow older.

PARENTS AND THEIR ADULT CHILDREN

Parents often assume that their children will grow up to have aims and convictions that are similar to their own. They may feel disappointed if their offspring decide not to follow in their footsteps. Points of conflict can include education, careers, religion, politics, and choices of friends, lovers, and marital partners.

Teenagers and young adults often want to distance themselves from their parents and lead different lives. They can also become angry at their parents, often years later, for the way in which they were brought up. Grievances that have been nursed silently for a long time may suddenly erupt when a child leaves home and discovers a new way of life. In extreme cases, parents and children may disagree on practically everything, leading to anguish for all.

Whether or not parents come to accept their children's choices, or the children become reconciled to the way in which their parents have chosen to live their lives, it is vital to keep the lines of communication open, especially if there are grandchildren involved. The relationship between a grandparent and grandchild is a very special one. It can bring stability and extra attention to the life of a child with busy parents, and great joy and pleasure to the grandparents. It would therefore be an enormous mistake to jeopardize this through anger over past acts or differences of opinion.

As long as parents and children continue to communicate in some way, there is a chance for them to work toward the future. Time does heal to some extent, but it may take some self-examination to see that the anger you are harboring is hurting you as much as it is an aging parent or adult child. Expressing your feelings in a nonaggressive way (see page 72) can help take the sting out of old wounds, and clear the way for a more satisfactory relationship.

SIBLINGS

Many brothers and sisters who were close as children remain so in adulthood. Others become closer as they grow up, leading to emotionally rewarding relationships as adults, not just for themselves but also for their families. Some siblings, however, find it hard to forget childhood rivalries, whereas others cannot come to terms with long-standing disagreements, where the slights and feuds of childhood have left scars that have not healed. Such simmering feelings can make family gatherings very tense, awkward, and stressful.

Although it may be hard to initiate the conversation, talking through problems that have existed since childhood with your brother or sister can be therapeutic. It might also be revealing, and possibly very funny, to share perspectives on some events that occurred when you were both very young.

If you have difficulty in reopening contact with a sibling, you might start with small gestures, such as sending a birthday card, or making a telephone call about something practical such as getting your mother's car fixed. Be patient and try to repeat similar gestures regularly, and in time you may reap the benefits of a much closer relationship.

GRANDPARENTS

Senior citizens today do not always conform to the popular image of the dear old grandpa and grandma, relaxing in rocking chairs. Many modern grandparents have their own interests, careers, and needs, and may not be available to help their offspring as much as their counterparts did in years past—filling in as baby-sitters, for example, or helping out with financial difficulties. Grown children have to recognize this and, while maintaining as much contact as is practical, they must understand that their parents have their own lives to lead.

Eventually, however, older members of the family may become frail and require special care. Losing independence because of declining health can be upsetting to people who, finally freed of their work and family responsibilities, have had a relatively short time to enjoy their new status in life. Elderly relatives can become depressed or morose and difficult to get along with when this happens. Family members can help by keeping in touch and showing that they value the older person's opinions and company.

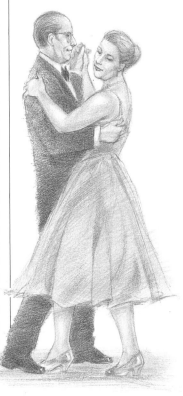

ACTIVE SENIOR CITIZENS
Today's grandparents are more youthful and independent, and are spending more time away from their families in pursuit of their own interests and hobbies.

The physical and mental deterioration of a loved one is extremely upsetting, and it may also be a source of guilt, especially if you live far away or work long hours and therefore cannot help as much as you would like. Hard choices may have to be made. Choosing a nursing home for an elderly person is especially difficult, even when it seems like the only option. Alternatively, a son or a daughter may decide to give up work and take care of a parent, which in itself can give rise to unforeseen strains and problems. The views of the elderly people as well as the demands of prospective care givers must be taken into consideration before any decision is made.

DISTANT RELATIVES

When family members live far apart, perhaps even reside on different continents, visits may be infrequent. Getting together with relatives you haven't seen in some time can be fulfilling but also stressful, as you may all be virtual strangers to each other and perhaps have very different outlooks and habits. When you don't know what to expect, it might be better to make a limited visit. If you plan to stay longer than a day or two, you should consider staying in an hotel. This will allow you to call on your relatives for a meal or to go on an outing, but not be with them for the whole time.

Try not to visit only at times of crisis, such as the illness or death of a family member. Your relatives will appreciate that you are making the effort out of a sense of duty, but they may also feel that you have no interest in seeing them for themselves. Moreover, visiting during a crisis may be more stressful to them than helpful.

You may not want to see relatives you have little in common with, but you could be pleasantly surprised by how a shared ancestry can forge a bond between you. You might also gain interesting new insights about your parents, siblings, or yourself.

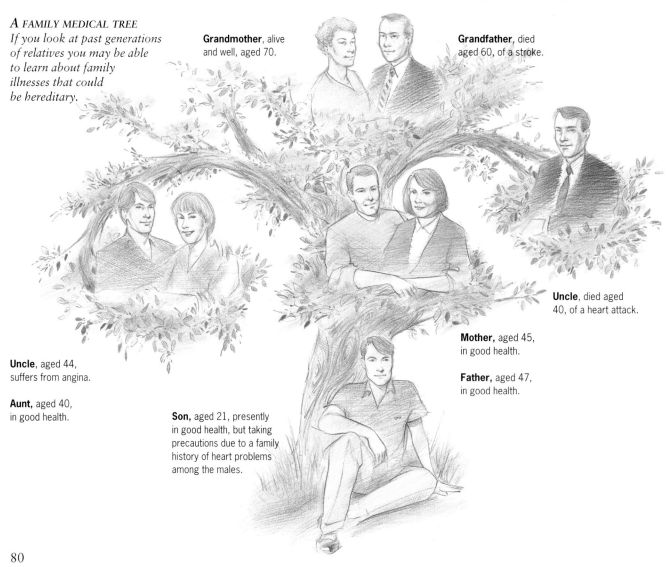

A FAMILY MEDICAL TREE
If you look at past generations of relatives you may be able to learn about family illnesses that could be hereditary.

Grandmother, alive and well, aged 70.

Grandfather, died aged 60, of a stroke.

Uncle, died aged 40, of a heart attack.

Mother, aged 45, in good health.

Father, aged 47, in good health.

Uncle, aged 44, suffers from angina.

Aunt, aged 40, in good health.

Son, aged 21, presently in good health, but taking precautions due to a family history of heart problems among the males.

RELATIONSHIPS AFTER DIVORCE

A marriage breakup is highly stressful, not only for the individuals concerned but also for their immediate families; and it can have serious effects on the couples' wider circle, including colleagues and mutual friends. But the most profound effect of divorcing parents is on the children. Suddenly their world is changed completely as they lose all their former stability. Often the first emotion they experience is panic, swiftly followed by fear of abandonment, anger, and powerlessness. Even though the parents themselves are experiencing great emotional turmoil, they must allow their offspring to express their feelings without overreacting to them. Because children are often very sensitive during times of family upheaval, it is best to treat them as gently as possible.

Youngsters can become very trying as they come to terms with a divorce, engaging in behavior that ranges from babyishness to aggression and rudeness, or withdrawal. If you understand that this is normal, and are patient but continue to set limits firmly, their adjustment will be easier. This phase can last for many months, and you too will be making adjustments, so it is important to have some support from friends or family, or even your family doctor.

Some children feel that the divorce is their fault, so it is extremely important that the circumstances of the breakup are explained to them in language they can understand. Children must be reassured that their sense of guilt has no basis in fact, and that you in no way blame them.

Except in the case of an abusive partner, the absent parent should be encouraged to maintain contact with the children. Some absent parents believe that their children are better off without them, but in fact they are important both personally and symbolically to their offspring. For children to be (or appear to be) rejected by a parent not only deprives them of someone to receive hugs and support from, but also could signify to them something deeper and more hurtful. At the very least, a parent's absence should be explained to children by the person concerned, and their birthdays and other special occasions should be marked by sending cards and gifts. The parent who has full-time care of the children should encourage this contact, which will have great significance for them.

When children are cared for by only one parent, it is common for them to lose touch with the family and friends of the other. But it's vital to maintain children's links with relatives and friends on both sides; otherwise they lose much more than a parent.

It will reduce your children's embarrassment if you tell other people, such as their friends' parents and perhaps their teachers, that you are getting divorced. This way the children do not have to break the news to others themselves.

REMARRIAGE

A second marriage can be a cause for joy, but it can also complicate an already overcharged emotional situation. For example, parents may have to learn to accept a son's new wife, even though his former one is still much loved and is the mother of their grandchildren. Brothers and sisters, too, may be hostile to the new partner and favor the previous one.

Children may frequently feel that they are helpless in the face of remarriage, when they have to become part of an instant family with none of the familiarity and shared history of their past one. They may also feel jealous of their stepparent and any stepbrothers and sisters, possibly seeing them as usurping their place in their parent's affections. As a result, children may misbehave, disrupting efforts to form a new family bond. Children can also feel a conflict of loyalty between the parent they live with and the absent parent and his or her new partner. This can be exacerbated if either (or both) of the parents criticize the other to the child. Divorced parents need to talk to their children as positively as they can about each other, and obey the golden rule, which is never to speak badly of the absent parent.

The role of stepparent can also be daunting for adults who have had little experience in living with or taking care of children. A relationship must be built gradually on mutual interests and trust, rather than trying to compete with the existing parent-child relationship. In any case, children need lots of understanding from the parents and their new partners at a time when the adults are trying to make their own relationship work. Even with constant reassurances of love and carefully negotiated rules, it may take time, patience, and hard work for the new state of affairs to be accepted.

Using positive reinforcement

If you have to reprimand your children, make it clear that it is their behavior you are criticizing, not them personally. Say, for example, "I am unhappy that you broke the china plate," rather than "How could you be so stupid?" Try to be rational and do your best to maintain a sense of humor.

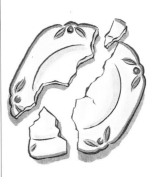

MAINTAINING PERSPECTIVES
Broken dishes can be mended or replaced, but a child's damaged feelings cannot.

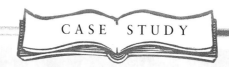
A Death in the Family

The death of someone you love—especially if it is unexpected—is a traumatic and stressful event. Dealing with it can be especially difficult if you don't know how to show your grief. Many health-care professionals believe that expressing your feelings is essential for good health, and that bottled-up emotions can manifest themselves as physical symptoms.

Forty-five-year-old Maureen was at work when her husband, Jim, was rushed to the hospital after a heart attack. She quickly realized that the attack was a serious one, and Jim died shortly after she reached his side. At first she felt only shock and disbelief. Both her daughters, Vicky and Clare, lived out of state, and during the first few hours after Jim died she felt too numb to contact them; the reality of Jim's death seemed unfathomable.

Soon after returning to their empty house, Maureen felt strong enough to break the news to the girls, and after a sleepless night, she started dealing with funeral arrangements. She thought she was not doing this well, but was relieved to have something to do. She imagined that people seemed embarrassed by her situation, so she kept conversations short.

Her daughters flew in to be with her, but as the funeral approached, they became withdrawn. Following the funeral, at which she cried very little, Maureen realized how angry she was with Jim for abandoning her. He had provided for her financially, but had left a chasm in her life. She also felt guilty that perhaps she hadn't helped him take care of his health, and she worried about her daughters, who remained distant with her. Maureen felt that life was not worth living.

Six months later, she was still very depressed. Frequently tearful, she was sleeping poorly and had little appetite. She was also neglecting her physical appearance, was paying bills erratically, and was often ill with minor complaints. Her work was suffering and she sometimes burst into tears. She knew this behavior was upsetting to colleagues, which made her even more distressed.

WORK
It can help to have a job to go to when there is a crisis at home, but your concentration may not be good.

HEALTH
Following a death in the family, the physical and emotional symptoms of grief can pose a health hazard for a year or two.

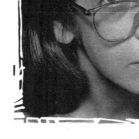

FINANCES
Even when provisions are made, taking sole responsibility for future finances might suddenly seem overwhelming to the surviving partner.

FAMILY
Communication can be difficult when everyone is unhappy, as family members are unable to share their grief.

BEREAVEMENT
It can take a long time to recover from a partner's death, especially if you keep your grief and resentment bottled up.

WHAT SHOULD MAUREEN DO?

Maureen needs to move on in the mourning process and help herself and her daughters come to terms with their loss. The four stages of grief—shock, anger, depression, and acceptance—are not always clear cut. Maureen should understand that not only is it normal to alternate among them, but also the process of healing can take a very long time, depending on the nature of the relationship, circumstances of the death, and the extent to which an individual is able to express grief.

It would help Maureen if she could find support from a trained outsider, such as a counselor, her family doctor, or minister. She should also talk with her daughters and encourage them to communicate their feelings to her. Expressing how deeply you have been affected by someone's death is an essential part of recovering from that loss, and the grieving process should not be rushed. Nevertheless, it is vital that Maureen start to think about all the other aspects of her future, including her health, work, finances, and social life.

Maureen needs to explain to friends and work colleagues that she is still grieving. This will help them to understand and accept that she is not her normal self. A support group for the bereaved may also help.

Action Plan

BEREAVEMENT
Have the family doctor recommend a professional counselor to help deal with feelings. Consider joining a self-help group for the newly bereaved.

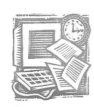

WORK
Talk with boss—perhaps he or she might be willing to delegate some duties to others. Explain difficulties to colleagues so that they can appreciate and make allowances for any lack of concentration at work.

FAMILY
Talk to Vicky and Clare about their father and try to bridge the gap that has opened up between them. Heart disease can have family implications, so the girls may need medical advice regarding diet and lifestyle.

HEALTH
Seek help for long-lasting depression. Get some advice from a doctor on taking better care of her health in general, and look into various relaxation therapies, such as yoga and meditation.

FINANCES
Gather together all bills, check books, and bank statements to determine financial situation. If necessary, make an appointment with an accountant to discuss handling affairs in the short term.

HOW THINGS TURNED OUT FOR MAUREEN

Maureen went to the bereavement counselor recommended by her doctor. At the sessions she talked about her anger with Jim for dying, how helpless she had felt at the hospital, and how inadequately she had coped with her daughters' grief. She and the counselor discussed ways to put her life back together and improve communication with her children.

She invited the girls home for the weekend and told them how she felt about what had happened; she also apologized for not having been as supportive as she thought she should have been. This opened the floodgates; both daughters openly wept about their father and talked about their own emotions. Grieving together as a family proved to be therapeutic and brought them closer together.

Maureen found the idea of talking to her friends and colleagues about Jim's death daunting, but once she raised the subject, she discovered that most of them were extremely caring and sympathetic. Some also gave her useful advice, putting her in touch with a support group for the bereaved, and also with an accountant.

Maureen began to eat properly for the first time in months, choosing foods to build up her strength. She and a friend began swimming once a week, and she also signed up for a yoga class. She found that the exercises relaxed her and the meditation healed her mind.

Today, although she still misses Jim terribly, Maureen is seeing the future as less bleak and is feeling much more positive about life.

THE COUPLE

Building and maintaining a long-term relationship takes work, patience, and compromise. A major factor in this process is open and continuing communication to prevent a build up of tension.

INITIAL ATTRACTION
In a US survey* of factors that initially attracted 890 men and 928 women to their future spouses, the number one factor, personality, also turned out to be extremely important in sustaining that attraction.

FACTORS	MEN	WOMEN
Personality	48	43
Looks	27	16
Warmth	13	25
Sexiness	8	8
Humor	1	4
Power	1	3

* The Janus Report on Sexual Behavior (Wiley, New York, 1993)

The majority of people marry, and many do so more than once; fewer than 8 percent of American women never marry at all, and only 9 percent of British men remain unmarried by the age of 40. But these days people are divorcing readily—one in every two couples in the United States, the United Kingdom, and Germany (see page 78).

The reasons that some couples stay together while others divorce are complex. Physical attraction is important, but personality and circumstances also play a part. In *The Janus Report on Sexual Behavior*, both men and women rated personality as the most important factor in initial attraction. It also seems to be the glue that holds a relationship together. In 1985, two American researchers, Jeanette and Robert Lauer, found that both women and men attributed the success of their long-standing marriages to their spouse being their best friend.

Even within the happiest relationship, however, the potential for conflict always exists. After the wedding, the first hurdle may be coming to terms with differences in the couple's expectations of marriage versus the reality. Later, the challenge may be to try to devise an equitable way of living when children arrive; and all relationships have to contend with the different backgrounds, personalities, habits, work, and social lives of the two people involved.

MAKING IT WORK

Above all else, if a couple is to have any chance of a successful, lasting relationship, they need to communicate with each other. Unfortunately, it is all too easy to fall into a pattern where confidences and worries are not shared and solutions are not worked out to suit both of the partners.

It is important to reconnect every day with your spouse. Even if you can manage

---

REFLEXOLOGY FOR COUPLES

Reflexologists treat ailments of the body by massaging "reflex areas" of the foot. But couples can also use foot massage to promote relaxation and reduce stress, by easing tense areas, and at the same time increasing intimacy.

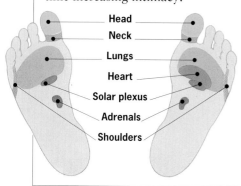

- Head
- Neck
- Lungs
- Heart
- Solar plexus
- Adrenals
- Shoulders

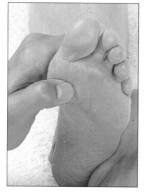

NECK POINT
Massage the ball of the foot up to the first joint of the big toe to relieve neck tension.

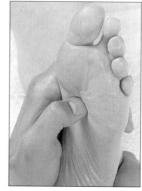

SOLAR PLEXUS POINT
Massage just below the ball of the foot in line with the second toe to ease emotional tension.

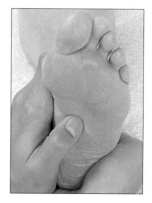

ADRENALS POINT
Rotate the thumb gently up and down the arch of the foot to relieve backache.

only five minutes of focused conversation, this will help you lessen any emotional distance that might have developed over the previous day. If both your lives are very busy, schedule a specific time at least once a week when you can sort through events and problems of the past few days and discuss the future. Try to do this away from your children, friends, and relatives.

Couples often shy away from discussing touchy subjects, just to keep the peace. For the sake of long-term harmony, it makes sense to deal with problems sooner rather than later, when they might be much more difficult to resolve. But it's important also to choose the right moment—no one wants to discuss difficult issues just after arriving home from work or when everyone in the family is hungry and wants dinner.

When the time is right, tell your spouse what is bothering you. To set a tone of goodwill, preface your remarks with a statement such as "I want to bring up something that's not easy for me to talk about." In fact, to avoid putting your partner on the defensive, always use "I" statements, such as "I feel angry when you do not wash the dishes," rather than, "You make me angry when...." Avoid sentences that begin with "You never..." or "You always...."

Remember that one of the joys of an intimate relationship is the freedom it gives you both to talk about anything. It also gives each of you more autonomy within your relationship, and provides a safe way to vent angry feelings that have nothing to do with the partner but can build up and lead to an explosion.

In modern Western society, it is common for couples to lead relatively separate lives, with both partners employed at different places or one taking responsibility for child care while the other works outside the home. If this is the case in your marriage, talk to each other about what you are doing and the people you come into contact with during the day. After all, what happens while you are away from each other—a car that will not start, for example—will undoubtedly have an impact at home. If this is too difficult, and you find yourselves drifting apart, try to find some activity that you can do together, such as playing tennis or bridge, gardening, or taking dancing classes, that relieves some of the stresses and strains of both home and work.

THE GLUE THAT MAKES A MARRIAGE STICK

In a 1985 survey*, 315 couples who had been married longer than 15 years gave their views on long-term relationships. Significantly, the first seven reasons given by each for a successful marriage were identical. They are listed here in descending order.

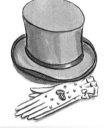

MEN AND WOMEN

▶ My spouse is my best friend.

▶ I like my spouse as a person.

▶ Marriage is a long-term commitment.

▶ Marriage is sacred.

▶ We agree on aims and goals.

▶ My spouse has grown more interesting.

▶ I want the relationship to succeed.

MEN

▶ An enduring marriage is important to social stability.

▶ We laugh together.

▶ I am proud of my spouse's achievements.

▶ We agree on a philosophy of life.

▶ We agree about our sex life.

▶ We agree on how, and how often, to show affection.

▶ I confide in my spouse.

▶ We share outside hobbies and interests.

WOMEN

▶ We laugh together.

▶ We agree on a philosophy of life.

▶ We agree on how, and how often, to show affection.

▶ An enduring marriage is important to social stability.

▶ We have a stimulating exchange of ideas.

▶ We discuss things calmly.

▶ I am proud of my spouse's achievements.

▶ We agree about our sex life.

* Survey by J. & R. Lauer, published in *The Janus Report on Sexual Behavior* (Wiley, New York, 1993)

LEARNING ABOUT YOUR SPOUSE

It is always worthwhile to keep up real communication with your partner. Talking, of course, helps, but if it only involves topics such as who is going to take the children to the dentist or how you are going to pay off that loan, you will not achieve the depth of intimacy that makes a truly satisfying relationship. Do not assume that you can read your spouse's mind; too many couples find out too late that they never really knew what each other wanted.

To learn another's innermost thoughts, it often helps to reveal some of your own first. This creates an atmosphere in which disclosure will feel welcome and safe. Something trivial, such as bringing up an embarrassing moment you had as a child, can then build up to more serious revelations.

It is important to listen actively to your partner when he or she begins to open up. Concentrate on what is actually being said,

TACKLING DISAGREEMENTS

A few practical changes in the way you communicate with each other can help defuse conflict.

▶ *Encourage your partner to give his or her view of events.*

▶ *Try not to make your partner feel guilty, and do not dredge up past mistakes.*

▶ *Even if you believe that you are totally in the right, accept some of the blame for the problem.*

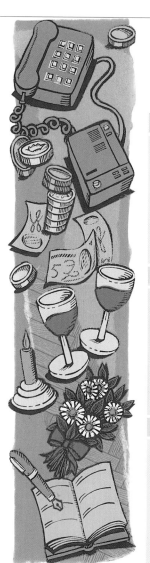

not on what you think about the statements or how you should answer. Don't tell your partner how to feel. Instead, just accept the other person's feelings.

If your spouse resists your efforts, respect his or her need for privacy. Some people find it extremely hard to talk intimately. You can, however, explain that the lack of intimacy in your relationship is difficult for you. Under such circumstances, you should make sure that you have someone you can confide in, because everyone needs intimacy in order to lead fulfilling lives.

Never try to find out more about your spouse's thoughts through such underhanded methods as reading a diary, opening mail, or listening in on telephone calls. You may misunderstand what is written or said, and if you are discovered, you could justifiably be accused of betraying trust. This would also be true if you were to use a confidence against your partner at a later date. If, for instance, a teacher confesses to her husband that she is having problems with her supervisor, and then during a later argument, he shouts: "See, you can't get along with anyone!" she is not likely to confide in him about future problems.

BRIDGING THE LANGUAGE GAP

Studies have shown that in general men and women differ considerably in their communicating styles. Deborah Tannen, Professor of Linguistics at Georgetown University in Washington, D.C., has pinpointed ways in which conversation between a man and woman can cause conflict.

Many men believe that in most areas of life, including communication, they must win over someone else to get what they want.

ACHIEVING CONNUBIAL BLISS

Today it is common for both spouses to have careers. When work stresses are added to those of communicating with each other and caring for a home and children, the result can be tension. Here are some ways to cope with the pressures.

ADD A ROMANTIC NOTE

No matter how busy you are with work and family demands, you should reserve some hours each week to be alone. The goal is simply to enjoy each other's company, rather than spending all your time discussing everyday problems. Keep your romance alive by giving your partner a suprise kiss or hug, bringing home a bottle of champagne, planning a special dinner, or organizing a weekend away.

PRIORITIZE GOALS

Decide together what are the most important things in your lives as a couple, but also as independent people. That way, when you are overwhelmed by conflicting demands you will be able to prioritize accordingly. Remember, it is all too easy to let life control you, rather than you controlling your life. If you know what you want and what will make you and your partner happy, then go for it.

CHANGE FOR THE BETTER

All relationships have room for improvement—all you need is motivation. To do this, both partners should make lists of all the things that annoy them—these can be major, such as spoiling the children, or minor, like never putting clothing in the laundry basket. Compare lists, then draw up another list, this time of how things could be changed. Work your way through it slowly, reinforcing changes as you go along.

DIVIDE CHORES EQUALLY

Look at who is responsible for what in your household. In a 1986 study, 74 percent of American couples rated equality in the relationship as important but it is not uncommon for a wife who holds a job to be responsible for most of the housework and child care. It is thus hardly surprising if she resents her husband. The ideal is to divide the work more equally, or if you can afford it, hire outside help.

SETTLE MONEY MATTERS

Decide how much money you actually need in order to live comfortably. Together you may be earning a lot, but to achieve this you may have to work at jobs that keep you apart or bring intense pressures into your lives. If this suits you, fine. But you might want to consider a simpler way of life, with perhaps less demanding jobs, so that you have more time for each other. Job sharing is one option.

COMMUNICATE—ALWAYS

The stresses of modern life can often render us speechless—with exhaustion. For this reason, most partners barely have the energy to speak to each other or, if they do, and they are both under pressure, they usually snap in irritation. This is not communication! To express what you want to say in a nonhurtful manner, always think before you speak and consider what the impact of your words will be on your partner.

Those who have this attitude usually feel more comfortable giving advice and orders than offering help and support, and they are frequently confrontational. Women, on the other hand, tend to regard communication as a means of achieving self-confirmation. They also desire intimacy, and usually prefer compromise to ordering people around or arguing with them.

These differing outlooks can cause unintentional hurt. Take the sentence "Let's go to the movies." A woman will typically regard this simply as a suggestion to agree to or not; a man may see it as an order and become angry. Or how about "Would you like to go to the movies?" A man, on being asked this, might weigh up the pros and cons in his mind, decide that he would prefer a night in, and decline the offer. His partner, on getting this response, might become upset because she was in fact, in a roundabout way, stating what she wanted to do and now feels that her desires are not being respected.

Different conversational styles can get in the way of honest communication, and so more directness on the part of women and more understanding on the part of men might go a long way toward bridging the communication gap. Without this, it is impossible for each person to understand what the other is getting at conversationally.

Achieving empathy

The power to identify mentally with others and understand them more fully takes conscious effort. The Native American saying, "Walk a mile in another person's moccasins" helps you to see yourself through another person's eyes.

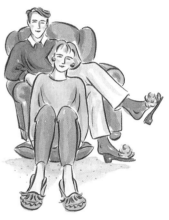

ANOTHER VIEWPOINT
It's important to put yourself occasionally in your partner's situation.

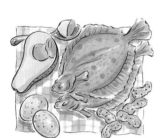

Whole grains, liver, fish, bananas, avocados, eggs, and potatoes are good sources of vitamin B_6, which may relieve some discomforts of premenstrual tension, and boost fertility.

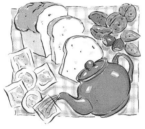

Nuts, whole grains, beans, and peas contain manganese, which may be involved in nerve function and fertility.

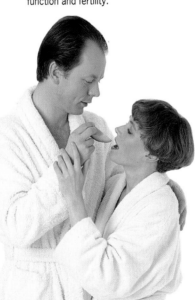

FOODS OF LOVE
Once the honeymoon is over, some couples find that sexual attraction wanes. Though oysters and champagne have been touted as the ideal food and drink for lovers, less expensive and more readily available ones may boost lovemaking and health.

Vegetable oils, nuts, seeds, margarine, and whole grains are rich sources of vitamin E, which may improve blood flow, strengthening a man's erection and also a woman's orgasm.

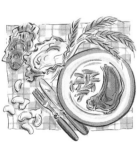

Meat, beans, oysters, milk, and whole grains are rich in zinc, which stimulates testosterone production, and aids sperm formation, erection, and ejaculation.

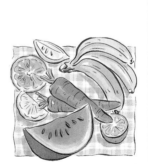

Green, yellow, and orange fruits and vegetables are rich in beta-carotene, which plays a role in the production of all sex hormones.

Sensuous Massage

Passionate relationships can become routine and predictable, particularly when people have been together for a long time. The physical side is often the first to suffer, but you can rejuvenate it with the power of touch.

SCENTED OILS

Essential oils can increase the sensuality of a massage, but be sure to mix them with a base oil—never apply them directly to the skin. Add them to your massage oil to enhance its effectiveness. For best results, 20 to 25 drops of essential oil can be added to a small bottle that contains about 2 fluid ounces (¼ cup) of base oil. This will usually be enough for one massage. To add atmosphere, heat oils in a vaporizer, or light an oil-impregnated candle.

An excellent way to enhance and bring new vitality to your sex life is to use massage for increasing feelings of warmth and intimacy. Massage also has the added benefit of helping to relieve physical and mental stress.

Simple massage strokes are easily learned and can be adapted to suit each partner's preferences. Seek feedback about the movements you use and listen to your partner—the massage is for pleasure.

You do not need to make any elaborate preparations. The essentials are privacy, warmth, subdued lighting, a suitable massage oil, and a supply of clean, soft towels. You will also need a firm, towel-covered surface to lie on. Most beds and couches are too soft to give adequate support for a massage, so you will probably have to use the floor. It can be made more comfortable by laying down an exercise mat, blanket, or a quilt.

SETTING THE SCENE

Careful preparation can turn a simple massage into a wonderfully sensual and erotic experience for both partners.

▶ *Lay out your towels and massage oil (or lotion) and turn the lights down low.*

▶ *Check that your fingernails are short, smooth, and clean.*

▶ *Take off any jewelry that might come into contact with your partner's skin.*

▶ *Ensure that you have absolute privacy and that the room is warm and free of any drafts.*

▶ *Have some gentle, atmospheric music playing in the background.*

▶ *Perfume the room with incense or a vaporized essential oil.*

* Do not use if you are pregnant.

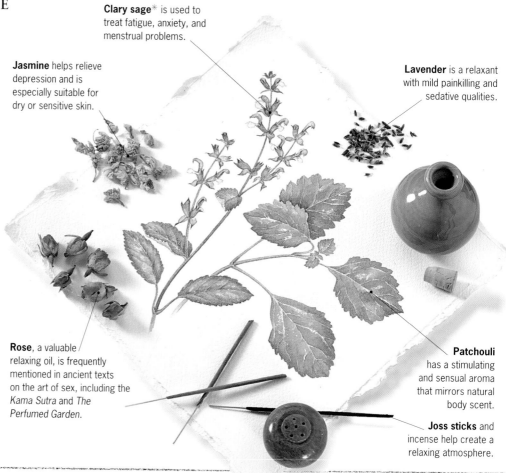

Clary sage∗ is used to treat fatigue, anxiety, and menstrual problems.

Jasmine helps relieve depression and is especially suitable for dry or sensitive skin.

Lavender is a relaxant with mild painkilling and sedative qualities.

Rose, a valuable relaxing oil, is frequently mentioned in ancient texts on the art of sex, including the *Kama Sutra* and *The Perfumed Garden*.

Patchouli has a stimulating and sensual aroma that mirrors natural body scent.

Joss sticks and incense help create a relaxing atmosphere.

Special oils and lotions, which help to reduce friction and make massage more sensual, are available from pharmacies and body-care shops. Grapeseed, sunflower, apricot kernel, almond, and soy oils are alternatives. Use an oil by itself, or enhance its effects by blending it with an aromatic essential oil (see page 68). For comfort, warm the oil by standing the bottle in hot water. Rub a little oil between both hands, then smooth it onto your partner's skin.

EXPLORING TOUCH

Another effective way to create intimacy, in addition to basic massage techniques, is by simply caressing each other all over, using delicate, fingertip strokes. You can combine this approach with massage or use it as an alternative.

Explore new touch sensations by stroking each other with sensuous fabrics, such as silk or velvet, soft, long-plumed feathers, or wooden massage aids.

CAUTION

Never give your partner a massage if he or she has: newly formed scar tissue; a skin infection, fever, or contagious illness; acute back or other pain; heart problems; thrombosis, phlebitis, or varicose veins; or any swelling or bruising.

MASSAGE STROKES

Take turns giving each other a massage. There is no correct sequence—use any or all of the following basic techniques, either spontaneously or in a more planned massage session. You can repeat each stroke as often as desired, but make sure you try new techniques to keep massage sessions exciting.

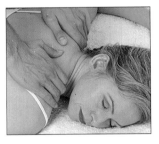

NECK AND SHOULDERS
With your partner face down, place a hand on each shoulder. Slide hands along shoulders and up each side of the neck, gently squeezing and releasing the flesh.

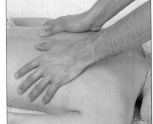

BACK
Using opposing circular strokes, move hands down the back to the buttocks. With fingers pointed toward the head, slide them firmly back up to the shoulders.

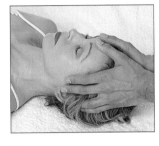

FACE
Gently trace your partner's face with your fingertips. Place your thumbs at the center of the forehead above the eyebrows; slide them out firmly toward the temples.

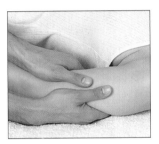

ARMS
With partner face up and palms on floor, stroke arms from wrist to shoulder with cupped hands. Work from shoulder to wrist, slide hands down inside of each arm.

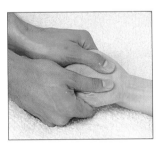

HANDS
Moving your thumbs in tiny circles, gently massage the fleshy areas of each of your partner's palms and the base of each thumb.

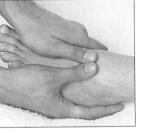

FEET
Stroke along top of each foot with your thumbs. Massage soles, moving thumbs in circular strokes.

LEGS
With your partner face down, stroke the back of each leg upward from ankle to buttock with cupped hands. Slide your hands back down the inside of the leg to the ankle. Ask your partner to turn over, and repeat strokes on the front of each leg.

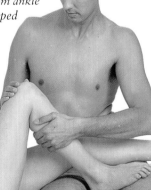

PARENTAL CONCERNS

Being a parent is enjoyable and rewarding, but it also brings its own stresses. There are some things you can do, however, to reduce the strain and make parenting more pleasurable.

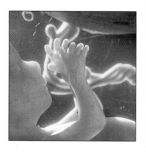

Fertility problems
For couples with infertility problems, anxiety can turn into anger, frustration, and loss of self-esteem, especially when friends start families without difficulty. Their stress is compounded by the tests that have to be performed before treatment begins, and increases during treatment, which not only disrupts their lives, but also has only a 35 percent success rate.

Changing from a couple to a family starts long before an infant arrives. Most babies today are planned, with couples often having numerous discussions before agreeing to go ahead. Some prospective parents make the decision easily, but then find pregnancy and the changes more problematic than anticipated. Still other couples, and in increasing numbers, find themselves unable to conceive. Both treatment for infertility as well as its failure can prove to be so emotionally damaging that a marriage may not survive.

Pregnancy itself is inherently stressful. A woman's body undergoes many changes—some are not always welcome—and the alterations in hormone levels can make her overly emotional. Prospective parents may become anxious about the new baby, and wonder what life will be like after the birth.

THE EXPECTANT PARENTS

A woman's health, financial situation, the stability of her marriage, and her job situation will work either for or against her ability to cope with the increased physical and emotional stresses of having a child. But whatever her circumstances, or those of her husband, learning more about the process of childbirth and child care will help the prospective parents to worry less. Many hospitals hold parenting classes, which include exercise and relaxation sessions for pregnant women, as well as classes that help her prepare for labor. Community centers may also have special exercise classes, and there is a wide range of literature available on all aspects of pregnancy and child care.

Many men delight in their partner's pregnancy, while others find it hard to cope with. They may be alarmed by the physical changes or feel shut out of the entire process. This can have a detrimental effect on the woman, who may feel that she has been left to face this major life change completely on her own. If this is the case, she should try to talk things through with her partner. If this fails, she should broach the subject with her doctor, who may be able to recommend the a counselor for help.

GREAT EXPECTATIONS

During pregnancy it's vital that partners talk to each other about how they feel. Although many men express a desire to participate in pregnancy and childbirth, it is not mandatory, and some women do not want partners to be involved. Each couple should come to an arrangement they're happy with.

IN TOUCH
A man can show his concern for his partner by minimizing her discomforts. Massaging her feet and legs can be very soothing.

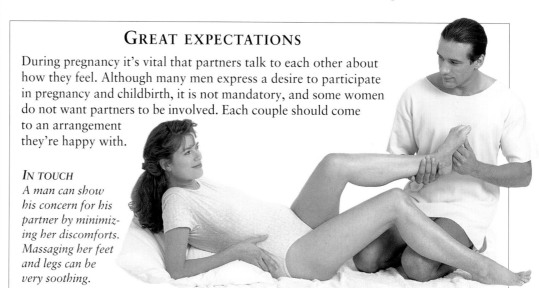

DID YOU KNOW?

Some men experience physical symptoms that mimic their partner's pregnancy and labor. Termed *couvade* by anthropologists, it is considered quite normal for men in certain tribes, such as the Chaorati of South America, to go through a false labor. More limited symptoms are commonly seen in Western men.

Individuals who experience the couvade are usually those who identify very closely with what their partners are going through. It should help such men to know that this is a well-known phenomenon, and that they can feel free to leave their partner's side during labor and childbirth if the events become too distressing for them.

POSTNATAL DEPRESSION OR BABY BLUES

A few days after childbirth, about two-thirds of all new mothers experience feelings of depression, when they cry or feel anxious for seemingly no reason at all. Called postnatal depression, or baby blues, this condition usually results from hormonal changes, and it generally disappears about two weeks after the birth of the baby.

Sometimes, however, these feelings last much longer. In environments that are supportive and geared to helping parents during this major life event, prolonged postpartum depression is virtually unknown, but throughout Western society at least 10 to 20 percent of all new mothers experience it.

There are certain stress factors that increase the chance of a woman becoming depressed after childbirth. She may have had an unhappy childhood or difficult relationships with her family. There might have been considerable medical intervention during the birth of her child, or the pregnancy may not have gone well. As a result, the woman could feel she has failed in some way. Conflict with the baby's father, financial worries, or loneliness are also possible factors. Fatigue and lack of sleep, combined with a baby that is difficult to satisfy, can make things even worse.

Most depressed women find that talking to a sympathetic listener is an enormous help. For a woman who is severely affected, professional counseling, drug therapy, or even hospitalization may be necessary.

BEING A GOOD ENOUGH PARENT

Many people today have little experience of childrearing until they have their own children. And if, as is the case for many parents nowadays, they don't want to raise their offspring as they were brought up, there are few rules to follow. Consequently, many new parents seek answers from the multitude of how-to books that purport to tell

Homeopathy after childbirth

A number of natural remedies are suitable to help a new mother. Discomfort of an episiotomy (cutting and stitching of the skin at the base of the vulval opening) may be eased by taking 30c Arnica four times a day until it subsides. The area can also be bathed in a solution, made by adding 10 drops of Calendula to 2 cups of water.

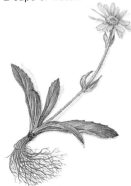

A SOOTHING CREAM
A cream containing Arnica and Calendula can be applied to sore and cracked nipples of breast-feeding mothers.

BABY MASSAGE

Massaging a baby from an early stage strengthens the intimate bond between parent and child and makes the baby receptive to physical touch. It also facilitates the relief of, and recovery from, many of the common illnesses that can afflict babies, including constipation, colic, coughs, and colds.

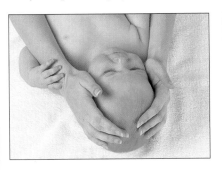

CRANIUM MASSAGE
With your palms, gently massage the crown in a circular motion. Then, using your fingertips, stroke down from the crown along the sides of the baby's face.

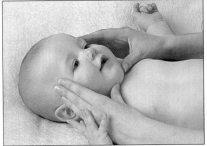

FACIAL RUB
With your fingertips, lightly stroke the forehead from the center to the temples. Then, using a circular motion, massage the baby's temples.

CHEST MASSAGE
Using both hands, gently stroke the chest from the center outward to the sides and back of your baby's body. Then gently stroke the diaphragm along the edge of the rib cage.

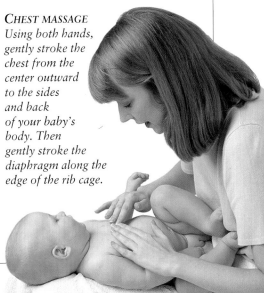

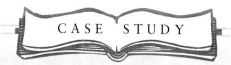
A Single Parent

Single-parent families have become common in Western societies. Most single parents are women, the majority of whom have to raise children with limited financial resources. This is stressful enough, but if the father withdraws his financial contribution as well as his affection, the consequences for the entire family can be shattering.

Diane has two young sons. A year ago, she and Eric, her husband of 13 years, divorced. Although she received regular alimony and child support from him for a time, both the money and his visits stopped when he was laid off. Diane is now receiving welfare, but it is not enough to feed and clothe two growing children and cover the usual household bills or any extras. Diane's savings are quickly becoming depleted.

The children are suffering too: the younger one has become withdrawn, and the older is becoming a bully. Diane always feels anxious and suffers from lack of sleep. She also lacks a social life and feels she will never enjoy herself again.

WHAT SHOULD DIANE DO?

To reduce the amount of isolation and helplessness she feels, Diane should seek assistance from her family and from other people in the community. To make her sons happier and provide a more stable environment, she must encourage Eric to see them and to cooperate with her for their benefit. At the same time, she has to make her sons see that none of what has happened between the parents is the boys' fault.

Diane also needs to obtain expert advice on getting the most out of her money, including all the benefits to which she and her family are entitled. Being able to relax would help her to sleep better and take a calmer view of her situation.

Action Plan

PARTNERS
Visit or telephone Eric to let him know how his absence is affecting his sons. Try to persuade him that seeing the children will benefit everyone.

FINANCES
Investigate free sources of advice. Ask social worker about benefits for which family is eligible.

HEALTH
Do something about feeling less anxious and getting more sleep. Join a single parents organization to get emotional support.

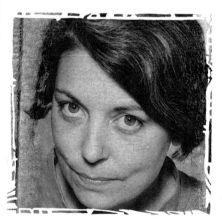

FINANCES
Welfare rarely covers a family's complete needs; money worries can prove to be the final straw to an overburdened parent.

PARTNERS
Many fathers stay away from their families after a divorce. This has grave consequences for the children as well as the mother.

HEALTH
Being on one's own with no one to talk to or share problems with can cause a parent to feel desperate and to act irrationally. Not getting enough sleep can lead to illness.

HOW THINGS TURNED OUT FOR DIANE

A librarian put her in touch with a single parents group and a yoga class. The former has enabled her to make new friends and meet potential baby-sitters, as well as providing advice on financial matters, benefits, and budgeting. The yoga class is free to mothers on welfare and has babysitting available for attendees. It took several phone calls to persuade Eric to see the boys, but he has; their behavior has now greatly improved, and so has the family's life as a whole.

inexperienced parents the "right" way to bring up their children. While offering much good advice, the authors of these books may differ in their opinions, often contradicting each other. There are really only a few basics required if you are to be what the psychoanalyst Bruno Bettelheim called a "good enough parent." Your children need love, security, consistency in the way you treat them, a modicum of discipline so that they know the boundaries of acceptable behavior, and most of all, they

UNDERSTANDING STRESSES ON CHILDREN

Stress can develop when youngsters covet certain material possessions that their parents can't afford or don't approve of, or when they feel pushed to achieve certain standards before they are ready. Parents should help their children develop a healthy perspective on the criteria by which they feel acceptable to others.

FAMILY POSSESSIONS

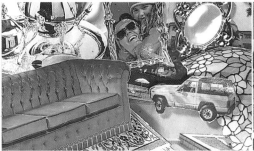

A house in an affluent neighborhood, with a pool or an expensive car, can place stress on a child who may feel that there is too much to live up to.

ATHLETIC AND SPORTING SUCCESS

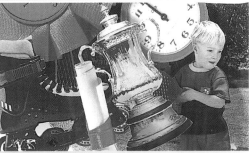

Being good at sports and winning awards and trophies can be gratifying, but it can also be a source of stress if a child feels pressure to repeat successes.

SUCCESSFUL PARENTS

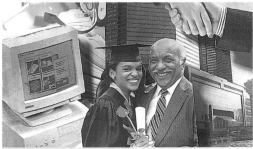

Having parents in a prestigious profession, or who are pillars of the community, may pressure a child to achieve academically or in a career.

SPENDING MONEY

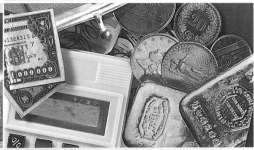

Earning one's own money is important but can be stressful if a child is not ready to take the responsibility of a job, yet desires financial freedom.

TRAVEL

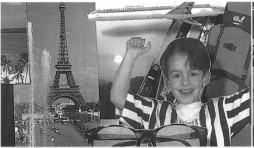

Exotic holidays are wonderful experiences, but children may feel that they need to have an expensive vacation every year in order to keep pace with their friends.

AUTONOMY

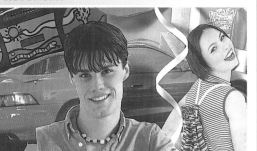

Perceiving that he has control and is free to make choices are vital to a child's maturity, but may lead to fears and anxieties about failure in the adult world.

Quality time

In the Western world an increasing number of mothers now work outside the home, at least 56 percent of those with children under the age of six and 73 percent of those with school-age children. Most psychologists agree that children of working mothers do not lose out. A study conducted in 1980 by a data-gathering service within the U.S. Department of Education showed that children whose mothers worked away from home read better than their classmates with stay-at-home mothers.

It matters less that you spend a great deal of time with your children than that the time you do spend is of sufficient quality. Give your child your undivided attention on a regular basis—if possible, an hour each day—for talking, playing, or reading together.

need communication. This is not to say that it is easy to be a parent (it can be very hard, for example, to be patient with a child who continually throws tantrums), but parents who keep the lines of communication open eventually reap the benefits.

Every family is different, so what problems arise and how you tackle them with your children will differ from the way your friends or relatives do. Parents' manuals should be read for pertinent advice, not taken as gospel. Talking with an experienced friend, your family doctor, a professional giver of child care, or even possibly a counselor can help you find solutions. You are not the first parent to have gone through these experiences, and this realization may bring you a measure of relief.

COPING WITH TEENAGERS
Because babies and young children are dependent on you, they are usually easier to deal with; also, you have control of their discipline. (They are, for example, small enough so that you can remove them easily from a difficult scene to be dealt with in private.) Teenagers are a different story. They are nearly adult size and can verbally and physically make your life truly miserable in their search for independence.

As youngsters grow older, they gradually become less dependent on their parents, forming a set of different relationships outside the family. Children between the ages of 12 and 15 have reached a pivotal point. On the one hand, they don't want their friends to see their dependence on their parents, but on the other they don't want their mothers and fathers to intrude on the identities they have forged for themselves among those of their own age group. Nevertheless, their need for parental reassurance—even if it is mostly unspoken—is still very strong.

The type and extent of the parents' discipline become crucial at this time: if it is too authoritarian, it invites almost rebelliousness, but if it is too lax, teenagers may regard this as evidence of the parents' indifference. According to experts in child psychology and family therapy, the most successful parents are those who manage to communicate their love and concern to their teenagers without being intrusive or overbearing. Limits are set, but these are gradually modified to give young people a feeling of independence.

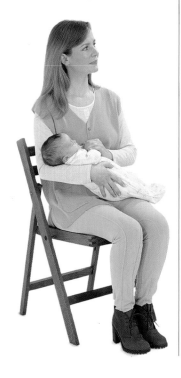

SELF-ASSERTION
New mothers can be inundated with offers of help or unwanted advice. To prevent arguments, convey your needs clearly to over-willing friends and family.

FAMILY VERSUS WORKING
Given that many of today's children grow up in dual-income households, the issue of child care can become a source of great stress in a marriage. Many mothers and fathers worry that their children will somehow become emotionally deprived if cared for by others, yet research has shown that good quality care can actually make children more independent and sociable. It can also, said American psychologist Alison Clarke-Stewart, even improve some children's educational levels. She found that children from poor backgrounds develop more quickly in day-care centers than they do when they stay at home, whereas children who are affluent develop at the same rate whether in day care or at home.

Often parents worry that by entrusting their child to a caregiver they will be losing touch during the important growing years, and that the children will be transferring their emotional allegiance to the caregiver. This is not so, because even if you work away from home, you will still spend more hours with your child in the mornings, evenings, and on weekends than any other person. Children are aware, from a very early age, that their mothers and fathers have a special status in relation to them, and they recognize that others have authority over them only because their parents have allowed it. Moreover, children have plenty of room in their hearts for a variety of close relationships; forming one with the person caring for them during the day can only give them an added sense of security.

But what kind of child care is best? In the United States at present, 35 percent of the children of working mothers are cared for by grandparents and other relatives; 20 percent are cared for by their fathers. While this option is more flexible—and less expensive—than day-care provision, it may cost more in terms of conflict and resentment in the family. For example, grandparents often have different perspectives on childrearing, and they may feel exploited if their goodwill is imposed on too frequently. Parents need to accept that they have delegated a certain amount of control and show appreciation.

Additional child-care options include other mothers, day-care centers and nursery schools, and nannies. When you consider employing people to look after your children, be very specific from the beginning about what you expect from them in the area of discipline, how the child should be occupied during the day, and how he or she is fed. It is also good to be very clear about the working hours, payment, what to do in emergencies, and so on.

Sharing the load

According to a British survey made by an insurance company, women in full-time employment spend an average of 49 hours a week doing housework in addition to their jobs. This imbalance can cause tremendous stress, because most women feel torn between the responsibilities and duties that are required of a wife and mother and those of a worker, regardless of whether they have careers or jobs soley for income.

It is therefore vital that you tell your partner as assertively as possible (see page 73) how you feel about this imbalance in the amount of housework being done by each of you. It may bring surprising and beneficial results. The same is true for children, who can be given increasing responsibility for small household tasks as they grow older. This is also excellent training for the time when they will leave home for good.

MANAGING TIME WELL

Dual-career families often find that it is nearly impossible to complete all of their housework, errands, and chores in the time available, which means that the hours set aside for relaxation disappear in a flurry of activity. Try some of the following ideas to help you organize your schedule and give you time for a rest.

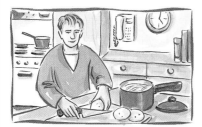

MEALS
To better organize food shopping and preparation, make a habit of planning menus a week in advance. If possible, use labor-saving devices, for example, a microwave oven to defrost and cook food quickly, and to fill the freezer, double recipes.

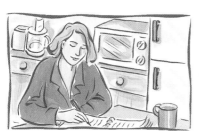

COMMUNICATION
To keep in touch with family members, get an answering machine. You can, for example, let them know about delays. Also, set up a bulletin board for schedules and memos.

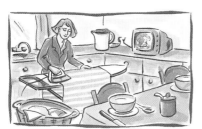

TASKS
To save time in the morning, set the table for breakfast after dinner. Also, lay out clothes needed for work the next day. Iron clothes in the evening before you go to bed or in the morning when you get up.

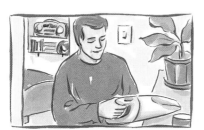

CLEANING
Distribute household chores to all family members; even small children can help sort laundry. Do a quick daily cleaning of bedrooms and living room, leaving larger tasks for the weekend.

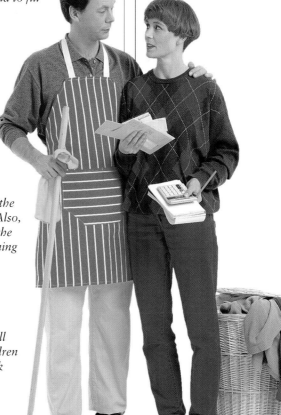

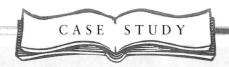
A Family Divorce

The breakup of a marriage is one of the most traumatic experiences that anyone can go through, and when children are involved, the problems multiply. Children often feel responsible for the split and need reassurance that they were not at fault. Parents must make an effort to deal calmly and fairly with what is at issue, so that a bad time can be made more bearable for all concerned.

During the last few years of their 16-year marriage, Joan and Bob were seeing less and less of each other, and they rarely talked of anything other than the children or the house. Both had careers, but Bob's took him away from home so often that Joan almost began to see herself as a single parent and to resent what she saw as Bob's jet-set lifestyle. Bob couldn't understand her anger: after all, it was his salary that allowed them to live in such a big house and want for nothing.

Everything came to a head when Bob suddenly announced that he had to go on an unplanned business trip and break his promise to see his son's play. As a result, Joan would not be able to attend a weekend management seminar that was vital to her career advancement.

This was the last straw. Bob must cancel the trip for the sake of both his son and his wife, or that would be the end of their marriage. When Bob refused and flew off on his trip, Joan had the locks changed and contacted a lawyer.

Joan felt both relieved and tense. She knew that it was hard to be a single parent, but she was almost one anyhow. The future, however, seemed very uncertain. She didn't earn enough to pay the mortgage and support the boys and herself.

Bob was outraged and bewildered. He had thought that his marriage, while not great, was more or less happy. He saw all that he had worked for going down the drain, and he was surprised to find how much he missed his sons. He decided to sue for sole custody of the children, as well as to keep the house.

Richard and Daniel, their sons, were shocked by this turn of events. They were used to their father's absence but still felt close to him. However, they recognized that their mother's complaints against their Dad were justified; at the same time, they worried that they themselves might have caused the break-up.

CHILDREN

If consulted, most children never want their parents to divorce. They often react badly, becoming withdrawn or aggressive.

FINANCES

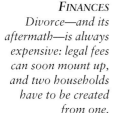

Divorce—and its aftermath—is always expensive: legal fees can soon mount up, and two households have to be created from one.

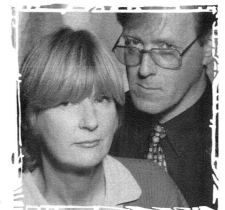

HEALTH

Divorce is a traumatic emotional experience that can sometimes result in mental and physical breakdown. The changed circumstances can cause the whole family to suffer.

PARTNERS

Whether one or both parties want the marriage to end, divorce usually leads to feelings of failure, a sense of betrayal, and great anger.

WHAT SHOULD JOAN AND BOB DO?

To settle their divorce with a minimum of bad feelings, Joan and Bob will have to put their emotions to one side while they sort out the legal and financial aspects of their future relationship. Anger and resentment can make sensible property, financial, and custodial arrangements difficult, if not impossible. Clear thinking and reopened lines of communication may not be a possibility without help from an uninvolved outsider (see box, below left), but they must agree that such help would be useful before they can progress.

Joan and Bob should stop arguing over the children and find a solution that takes into account their sons' points-of-view. It is imperative that they don't put the boys on the spot by making them choose one parent over another to live with. Joan and Bob must also make every effort to reassure their children that the divorce is not their fault; rather it is a result of their own relationship breaking down. The goal is for the boys to maintain a good relationship with both of their parents so that they feel secure in their love.

Action Plan

CHILDREN
Make legal agreements about custody of the children, living arrangements, and visitation rights. Bob must decide if he is really committed to working less so that he can look after his sons. Consult the boys about the situation and try to deal with their emotions as compassionately as possible.

FINANCES
Come to an agreement on child support and payments on the family home. Joan will have to ask Bob to help her manage the mortgage, or else consider moving somewhere more economical.

PARTNERS
Joan and Bob should talk individually to a close friend or relative who is a good listener. They should also attend mediation or ask the family doctor to recommend a professional marriage counselor.

HEALTH
Joan and Bob each need to consider some method of relaxation, such as yoga or meditation, to minimize stress. They should eat sensibly, resist smoking, and try not bury hurt feelings in alcohol or food.

MEDIATION

Independent mediation services are increasingly available for divorcing couples, and they are often recommended by experts in the divorce field. An impartial third party—a mediator—will meet with both partners and their children separately to discover their feelings and needs. The object is for the partners (and, if they are old enough, the children) to discuss these matters together in an informal, non-legalistic setting, so that they can come up with acceptable solutions. Mediation is not intended as a means of reuniting couples, but instead is aimed at helping them make considered decisions.

HOW THINGS TURNED OUT FOR JOAN AND BOB

Joan and Bob contacted a mediation agency and met with a mediator for six months. They found the process painful, but as they discussed their marriage, they realized that it really was at an end. They gradually found that they could express their regret and sense of failure.

After lengthy discussions, Bob realized that for practical reasons he would not be able to care for Richard and Daniel, but he did want to see them frequently. He and Joan agreed to sell the family home and share the proceeds; Joan would buy a less luxurious house and Bob an apartment nearby. He would pay child support for the boys, but she would carry the mortgage on the new house and support herself. The boys would have two homes: they would visit Bob on weekends, but would live most of the time with Joan. Bob told his sons that he thought it would be good for the three of them to take up a hobby; they decided to go windsurfing together.

To relieve anxiety and tension, Joan and Bob each tried a variety of relaxation techniques, including meditation, massage, and aromatherapy. Although initially traumatic, the divorce eventually had some long-term beneficial effects for all of the family.

Family Therapy

All families encounter problems from time to time. These may relate to one individual or to events over which the family has no control. Many can find solutions on their own, but some can benefit from the help of a trained outsider.

THE FAMILY AS A SYSTEM

Family therapy is also known as systemic family therapy because it holds that the emotional and pyschological relationships of a family act as a dynamic system. Although a single member of the family may often appear to be the "affected" individual, he or she is in fact simply acting as a scapegoat for disturbances in the whole family system. Thus a problem child's behavioral disorder, a common reason for families to attend therapy, is viewed as the expression of the whole family's problem.

Family therapists, or counselors, are trained in psychotherapy or counseling. They take a holistic approach—everything that happens to one member of a family must be considered in relation to the whole group, and everyone's opinion should be sought to find the best solution. They also believe that if traumatic or stressful events are not dealt with openly, family members will hide their feelings, which may erupt later in negative behavior that will ultimately affect the entire family.

What problems do family therapists deal with?

Therapists deal with a wide range of problems. The most common are relationship problems between family members; stress resulting from dual demands of home and career for adult partners; financial pressures; children who bully or are being bullied; children—often adolescents—who have other behavioral problems that affect the entire family; bereavement, separation, or divorce; the trauma of child abuse.

STAGES OF FAMILY THERAPY

Seeing the results of family therapy usually takes time and more than one meeting. Most therapists prefer that the entire family attend, because a problem with one or more members affects everyone. Sometimes, those who initially refuse to take part change their minds once they see that the others are benefiting.

1 *All family members feel nervous and uncomfortable. The therapist starts the discussion.*

2 *Trust is established and the therapist hears comments from all of the family members.*

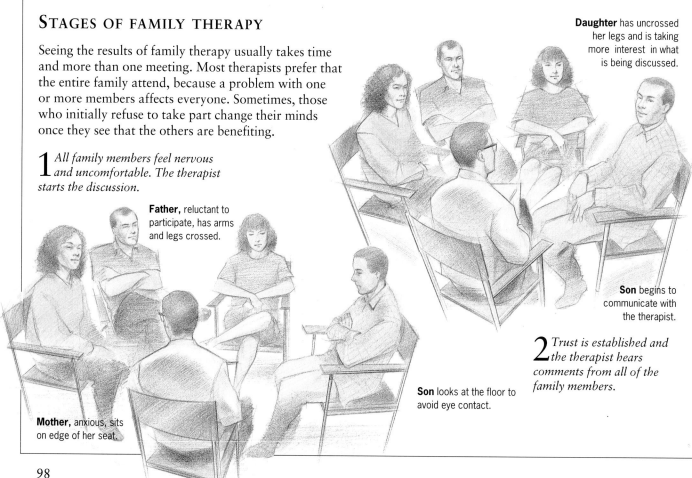

Daughter has uncrossed her legs and is taking more interest in what is being discussed.

Son begins to communicate with the therapist.

Son looks at the floor to avoid eye contact.

Father, reluctant to participate, has arms and legs crossed.

Mother, anxious, sits on edge of her seat.

What happens in family therapy?

During sessions, each person has the opportunity to state his or her viewpoint to the therapist in front of the rest of the family, and no one is allowed to interrupt. Some of what is said may seem ridiculous or be extremely hurtful; however, on reflection, many people find that the feelings expressed during these sessions have helped them to understand things that previously had puzzled or worried them about the relationships within the family.

What is the role of the therapist?

The role of the therapist is to ensure that everyone has his or her say, to guide the family toward tackling problem areas, and to control the situation if it becomes emotionally tense. The therapist will avoid passing judgment and will try to help the family look for solutions, come to their own conclusions, and make compromises where necessary. Then he will be supportive of whatever decision is reached.

How long will each session last?

A session normally will last from 45 to 50 minutes. This is usually sufficient time for each person to speak and for the therapist to initiate discussion, but not so long that the participants, particularly children, become emotionally exhausted.

How many sessions will be needed?

This varies with the type of problem. One session may be sufficient to open the floodgates for discussion on a previously taboo subject, such as the death of a loved one. For more long-standing or complex problems, however, it will probably take some time to unravel the emotions of everyone involved, and deal with them. As a rule, you should attend at least four sessions before making any assessment of their worth.

What does a family get out of going to family therapy?

During the therapy sessions, each member has the opportunity to speak freely and be listened to with respect.

Often, this is not possible at home, where only the person who is the most assertive or who has the loudest voice or the greatest authority is heard. Additionally, family members begin to gain perspective on their own role in the family; this insight will help them improve interaction.

How do I go about finding a family therapist?

Ask your family doctor to recommend someone who is properly qualified. Once you have checked a therapist's credentials, ask for a preliminary meeting to find out how the therapist will run the sessions, what the charges are, the sort of psychological philosophy he or she holds and—most important—if you feel comfortable with him or her.

WHAT YOU CAN DO AT HOME

Knowing how your behavior affects the members of your family is the first step to improving relationships and creating a happier and more harmonious atmosphere. It is very important that you gauge your response before you communicate it to others. This should help you to avoid unnecessary and potentially hurtful confrontations.

3 All family members have expressed their opinions and the therapist has guided them to some conclusions, thus helping to resolve the problem. Everyone is happier and more relaxed.

Mother displays physical affection toward her son.

Father and daughter are smiling, gesturing, and actively participating in the conversation.

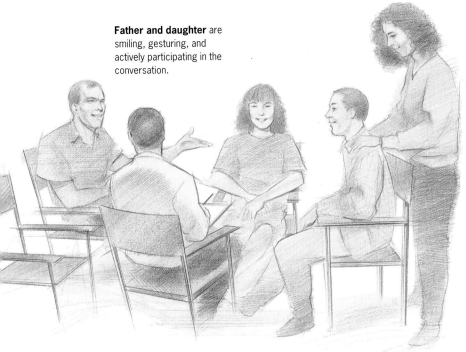

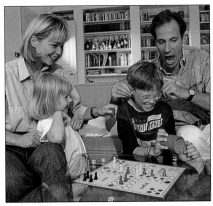

SPENDING TIME TOGETHER
Finding things of mutual interest to enjoy together is one way for a family to offset tensions and discover new ways of communicating effectively.

99

THE CHILDREN

Children under stress are often unable to express what they are feeling and may show that they are upset in indirect ways. They might become aggressive, for example, or physically ill.

ACCEPTING A NEW BROTHER OR SISTER

Although a new baby in the family is a joyful event, it can also threaten an older child. To help smooth the way:

▶ *Before the birth, start the older child in a play group or nursery school —something that only "big" children do.*

▶ *When the baby is born, give the older child a present from the baby, and devise special treats that are appropriate only for big boys and girls.*

▶ *Have a relative make the older child his or her special concern, to replace the temporary loss of the mother's attention.*

BEING A BIG BROTHER
Allow the older child as much contact with the newcomer as possible.

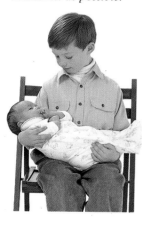

A child's relationship with brothers and sisters is immensely important, and often very rewarding and pleasurable. It can also, however, be a source of jealousy and rivalry. Some children become very clinging when a sibling arrives, so parents need to consider how to keep this to a minimum. The birth of a new family member frequently makes older children feel displaced, and they may respond by regressing to babyhood, perhaps wetting their beds, or becoming destructive as they play out their anger, or showing aggression towards the new baby or other children.

They need reassurance that they are still loved, and their feelings should be appreciated, not dismissed. If parents are disapproving or critical—saying, for example, "Don't be such a big baby."—children will hide their anger. This feeling could later emerge as intense rivalry towards, or even hatred of, the newcomer.

Another source of stress for children can be the way their families sometimes label them, calling them, for example, "the smart one" or "the pretty one." Parents should understand that children are more likely to thrive if they feel that all options are open to them for as long as possible, and they may feel stress if they have to fulfil other's expectations of them. Anxiety also can be caused if parents compare one child to another. If one child is less gifted than another, remember to praise him or her for something more general, such as good behavior or being helpful, and be careful to distribute hugs and kisses evenly.

SCHOOL DAYS
Children spend, on average, six hours a day at school, which for them can be a potentially stressful environment. A positive attitude on the part of their families will help them to settle happily in school. Parents

---

IS YOUR CHILD UNDER STRESS?

Any of the behaviors below may indicate that your child is under stress, especially if such behavior is prolonged. You can help by trying to get your child to talk

about his or her feelings. If, despite this, the unacceptable behavior continues, you should consult your family doctor or consider seeking professional help.

▶ *Exhibiting regressive behavior, such as bed-wetting, demanding to be bottle-fed, and throwing tantrums*

▶ *Refusing to go to sleep or having nightmares*

▶ *Being aggressive, unusually naughty, unruly, or destructive*

▶ *Stammering*

▶ *Refusing to eat*

▶ *Lying or stealing*

▶ *Being weepy, fearful, or clinging*

▶ *Refusing to go to school or skipping classes*

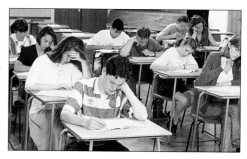

EXAMINATION PRESSURE
The stress of taking exams can, in extreme cases, lead older students to commit suicide.

DEALING WITH SOME COMMON CHILDHOOD PROBLEMS

AGE	CHILDREN WILL BE	PARENTS MAY BE	PARENTAL SOLUTION
0–1 (BABYHOOD) 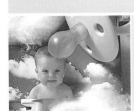	Learning to make sense of the world. Being sweet, charming, yet incredibly demanding. Crawling, with its potential dangers.	Exhausted from giving constant care and attention, compounded (in early months) by lack of sleep.	Take a nap or rest when your baby does. When crawling starts, baby-proof the house as much as possible by moving dangerous or breakable things out of reach.
1–3 (TODDLER) 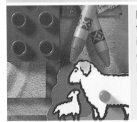	Learning to express themselves and be more independent, but feeling constant frustration. Having screaming fits and temper tantrums.	Stressed out in private and embarrassed in public by "terrible two's."	Develop organized routines so that your child has only a few new things to cope with. During a tantrum, distract him or her with an activity, toy, or story.
3–5 (PRE-SCHOOL) 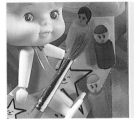	Venturing out. Anxious about starting school and making friends. Perhaps learning to accept a new baby in the family.	Concern for the child, wanting the best for him or her. Worried about his or her capabilities and whether you have provided good groundwork for learning.	Try not to overreact because you are worrying about your child's future. Believe in your child's ability to do whatever he or she wants, and provide lots of encouragement.
5–9 (SCHOOL-AGE) 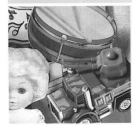	More independent. Taking no notice of you, rudely saying that you do not know anything. Acting out in school and hard to discipline.	Frustrated by child's growing independence but continual immaturity. Worried about child's adjustment to school and social life.	Listen to your child and consider his or her views seriously; try to deflect anger with humor. Be consistent and firm in your own views and behavior.
9–13 (ADOLESCENCE) 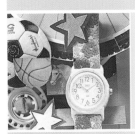	Embarrassed and confused about physical changes and feelings. Finding diificulties in trying to cope with the opposite sex on a social level.	Nervous and shy about discussing body changes and also sex. Perplexed by their youngster's moodiness and desire to be by himself or herself.	Talk directly to your son or daughter about puberty and sex. Be prepared to answer questions, even on disconcerting topics. Above all, be open and honest.
13–17 (YOUTH) 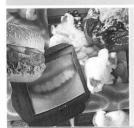	Considering future. Worrying about schoolwork, college, or employment. Struggling against parental restrictions.	Apprehensive for the future and safety of youngsters. Hurt and angered by disagree-ments and disruptions to family life.	Encourage your child to talk about his or her future. Emphasize studying but without pressure. Increase amount of freedom, with reasonable limits.

Getting children to sleep

Bedtime can become a battle of wills between parent and child, especially if the child is overtired or overexcited. Lavender oil has soothing, sedative properties, and the aroma from burning it may help calm your child or baby into sleep.

SOOTHING LAVENDER
A lavender-filled pillow, or one impregnated with lavender oil, can be a helpful remedy for insomnia.

Bullying

Bullying has become a major problem in schools. Children who are repeatedly harassed, verbally or physically, by other children lose their confidence and sense of security. Bullying also causes great concern for the parent. In extreme cases parents have been known to move so their child can attend a school in a different area. Bullying should always be reported to school authorities, many of whom are now developing policies to combat this problem.

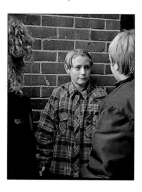

PLAYGROUND FEARS
Stress on a child , which is caused by bullying, can make school a place to be feared and have a negative impact on behavior at home.

should expect everything to be fine; if they show signs of anxiety, indicating that they think their child may be frightened without them, he or she will fulfill their expectations by becoming worried, too. Children can succeed at school when they are encouraged to regard it as a place where their parents are happy to send them.

Even so, your children are bound to suffer some stress from school. They may have problems getting along with teachers or classmates. Friendships may be quickly made and then hurtfully broken, signs of individuality might be rebuffed by classmates, and, once a child reaches high school, the competition for girlfriends and boyfriends can result in as many losers as winners. In addition, difficulties in keeping up with their coursework, and sometimes obsessive worry about exam results, can make high school a harrowing experience.

Parents should let children know that they are always there with a sympathetic ear. They must be careful, however, not to interfere unless asked to do so, as an intrusive parent can damage a young person's standing among his or her classmates and impact negatively on self-esteem.

It is also important that children be appreciated for themselves and their own abilities even if their achievements at school are only modest. Encouragement will ensure they

make the most of themselves, although there is a fine line between this and burdening them with unrealistic expectations that they cannot fulfill; parents need to be careful not to push too hard.

SERIOUS ILLNESS

When very sick, young children appear especially vulnerable, but in fact they often handle serious illness quite well. It is more frequently the parents who become traumatized. It will be helpful if you hide your own worries. Your child is likely to be frightened by unpleasant symptoms, and your calmness and control can be reassuring. You must be truthful, however, so the youngster will feel free to talk to you about any worries or fears he may have.

If a young person has to be admitted to a hospital and you have time to prepare, find books (picture books for the very young) that describe life in a hospital. You can use these to start a discussion about what is going to happen, which will go a long way toward allaying a child's fears. Some hospitals will agree to visits before the admission date so that a child can become at least a little familiar with this new environment, and many also allow one parent to stay with the child throughout an illness. These visits can be reassuring for both yourself and your child during what can be a stressful time.

THE ROLE OF FAIRY TALES

Small children tend to see the world in black and white, ignoring the confusing gray areas that are often beyond their comprehension. For example, a child may find it hard to reconcile the loving behavior of the parents with the anger and aloofness that they can exhibit, particularly when the child has been naughty. And even small children are not immune to the talk of violence and death that permeate every news broadcast.

Fairy tales offer a safe area in which children can work through scary notions such as being abandoned by their parents or attacked by strangers. The stories also allow them to be frightened of something outside their own small world, with the knowledge that in these special scenarios there is almost always a happy ending.

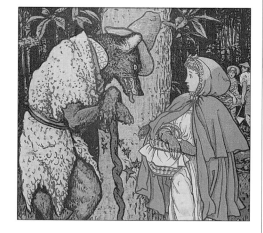

REASSURING RED RIDING HOOD
Children easily identify with the good and bad characters in popular fairy tales. You can use stories to help your children confront and overcome their own fears.

CHAPTER 6

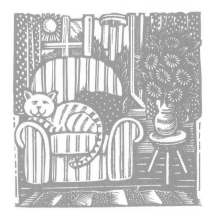

A STRESS-FREE HOME

*Your home should be the place where you
rest and recuperate from life's pressures, where
you can close the door against external stresses.
Many factors contribute to this haven—pleasing
colors and furniture placement, appropriate lighting,
pleasant aromas, and more. Vital, too, is safety within the house and the know-how to keep intruders
out. In this chapter we show you how to create
a safe and relaxing environment in every
room, and a welcoming atmosphere
for your family and friends.*

MAKING YOUR HOME A HAVEN

When your home is pleasing to the senses and is kept in good order, it can be a haven from stress, a place where you can relax and recharge your batteries in comfort.

A RITUAL FOR UNWINDING

You will feel more relaxed when you get home from work if you make a clear distinction between it and your workplace. To do this you could:

▶ *Put on your favorite music or television show.*

▶ *Take a hot shower or a long, soothing bath.*

▶ *Change your clothes and shoes to something more comfortable, and as different as possible from your work clothing.*

▶ *Treat yourself to a warming drink in winter, or an iced or cool beverage in summer.*

To make your home a calm center to your busy life, consider the effects not only of color and lighting, but also of sound, air quality, and odors.

COLOR AND LIGHTING

The colors in rooms can do much to create a certain mood (see box, opposite page). They also affect your perception of warmth and coolness, and can be used to offset the climatic condition which results from a room's position. For example, if you want to cool down south-facing rooms, which are normally sunny, furnish them in blues and greens. To warm up north-facing rooms, which are in shade much of the day, use reds, oranges, and yellows.

Your own reaction to certain colors is significant, too. Those that you like will make you feel good, wherever you use them. But you can have too much of a good thing. Rooms will generally be more soothing if you keep the walls and flooring in light to medium neutral tones and use favorite colors in upholstery, draperies, and accessories.

Lighting has a major effect on a room's color scheme (it can enhance it or make it seem drab) and on its mood. Each room in a home needs a variety of lights to achieve a pleasing effect and to suit different purposes

and activities. Background lighting, usually from a ceiling fixture, should illuminate the whole area with a low level of light. If there is no ceiling fixture, then you need two or three lamps to get a similar effect. Task lights must provide enough wattage to do a particular job, such as putting on makeup. Accent lights are used to call attention to a particular decorative element, such as a painting, tapestry, or sculpture.

Dimmer switches allow more flexibility in lighting. For instance, a dimmed ceiling fixture can set a soft mood for dining. The color of bulbs is important, too. Pink bulbs give a much warmer light than white; blue, even the light blue of some fluorescents, will create a subdued feeling.

SOUND

Unpleasant external noise can disturb not only your sleep but also your mental state when you are awake. If you live in a noisy neighborhood, consider investing in very thick draperies and double- or triple-glazed windows. If this is not effective enough, try to negotiate with neighbors about keeping noise levels down.

Some noises that bother you might be within your own control. For example, if your refrigerator is buzzing loudly, it may need repairing. If excessive noise emanates from your heating or air conditioning system, have an expert inspect it. And for noise that you cannot control, a good sound system playing your favorite music can mask much of the irritating background clatter.

AIR QUALITY

The air quality in your home can have a great effect on how you feel. If you are cold, your muscles will become tense; if you are

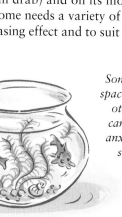

PET THERAPY
Some pets require more space and attention than others, but all of them can provide relief from anxiety, loneliness, and stress (see page 110).

hot, you may feel sleepy and lethargic much of the time. Experiment with various heating levels: altering temperature by just a few degrees can make a big difference.

If central heating has been drying out your skin and breathing passages, installing a humidifier is one solution. Another, less expensive way to solve the problem is to place shallow containers of water on radiators or hang them over heating vents. Potted plants also help to keep humidity levels more comfortable. Where high humidity is common in summer, hot weather can be unbearable. If you do not have air conditioning, one solution is to install a dehumidifier; another is to use fans. An attic exhaust fan is very effective for drawing out hot air.

SMELL

One sense often overlooked in a home is smell. The connections in the brain for it are closely linked with the circuits of the limbic system, which deals with emotion. This is why some scents bring childhood memories flooding back, and why a room, although perfect in every other respect, may feel uncomfortable if the smell of it is somehow wrong. Real estate agents sometimes suggest that their clients bake bread or make fresh coffee when prospective buyers are coming, as these aromas create an agreeable atmosphere.

There are many other ways to give your house an appealing smell. First, go outside

continued on page 110

COLOR IN YOUR HOME

Psychologists, artists, and decorators all know that color can be used to influence mood. For example, blue is the color of peace and communication and is suitable for rooms where you normally relax and converse. Green, which enhances concentration and creativity, may be a good choice for a study or workroom. Yellow and orange are welcoming, while red is sensual and stimulating. The more intense a color is, the more strongly its effects will be felt. Also, paler tints make a space seem larger, darker shades, smaller.

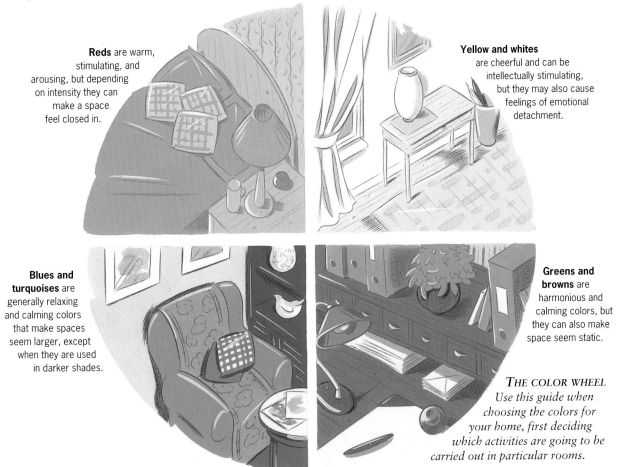

Reds are warm, stimulating, and arousing, but depending on intensity they can make a space feel closed in.

Yellow and whites are cheerful and can be intellectually stimulating, but they may also cause feelings of emotional detachment.

Blues and turquoises are generally relaxing and calming colors that make spaces seem larger, except when they are used in darker shades.

Greens and browns are harmonious and calming colors, but they can also make space seem static.

THE COLOR WHEEL Use this guide when choosing the colors for your home, first deciding which activities are going to be carried out in particular rooms.

105

Feng Shui

Feng shui is an ancient Chinese art that evolved from the observation that human beings are affected—positively or negatively—by their surroundings. Recognizing and respecting this can result in a harmonious and prosperous environment.

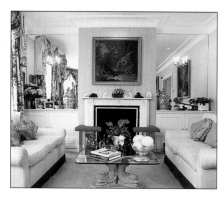

THE POWER OF FENG SHUI
Feng shui can be used to create a home where harmony reigns and beneficial energies are free to flow.

According to the masters who practice it, the aim of feng shui is to ensure that correct choices are made concerning the position of structures and objects. This, in turn, will alter the environment and harmonize it in a way that will improve the well-being and prosperity of those living and working in the space. The term feng shui means "wind" and "water," and it is held that these forces are responsible for determining health, wealth, and good luck.

While most people would recognize that a badly designed room, insufficient space, or a visually unpleasing shape may make them feel ill at ease, or that a poor choice in lighting or furniture may be uncomfortable, the exponents of feng shui carry this concept one step further. They believe that more than just an issue of esthetics or physical comfort, the design, combination, and positioning of objects creates a physical force in its own right, one that may act for good or for ill.

Who uses feng shui?
Feng shui can be applied to any size living or working space—from something as small as an office desk to an area as large as an entire country. The practice has many branches

FENG SHUI REMEDIES
Once feng shui masters have made their assessment of a space, they will suggest changes to remedy situations that are unharmonious. The following are frequently recommended:

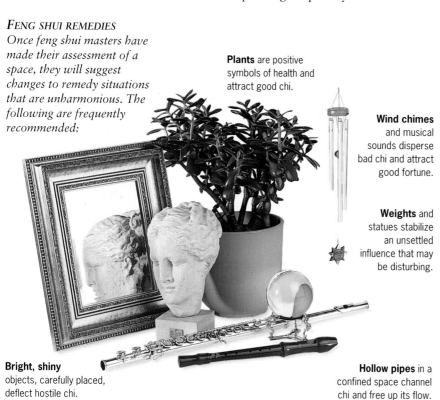

Plants are positive symbols of health and attract good chi.

Wind chimes and musical sounds disperse bad chi and attract good fortune.

Weights and statues stabilize an unsettled influence that may be disturbing.

Bright, shiny objects, carefully placed, deflect hostile chi.

Hollow pipes in a confined space channel chi and free up its flow.

Origins

Feng shui evolved from the agrarian way of life in China during the Shang dynasty (c.1766–1123 B.C.). Because farmers lived in an environment that was often hostile, they had to find ways of coexisting with nature in order to survive. Siting a farmhouse halfway up a south-facing hill might provide shelter from harsh winds and floods, and at the same time ensure enough sun for crops to grow. The Chinese in ancient times recognized the power of nature and the importance of harnessing it without interfering with or exploiting it. If nature is treated respectfully, they believed, it will yield power and prosperity.

and a wide range of applications. Masters train for a number of years, and their expertise is employed not only in private homes, but also in industry and government.

How does feng shui work?
The art of feng shui is based on the observation and understanding of *chi*, the life force that—practitioners believe—exists in all living things. Positive chi is said to be responsible for good health and spirits. For this reason, much of Far Eastern philosophy and medicine is geared toward balancing chi. A feng shui expert looks at the ways in which the impact of a space can be enhanced to produce more positive chi.

Feng shui's goal is to tap the earth's chi, just as the role of acupuncture is to tap a person's chi. According to the feng shui masters, buildings, trees, even sunlight affect the quality and flow of chi. Their aim is to create a place where chi flows smoothly and the principles of yin and yang are balanced.

What do feng shui masters do?
Central to feng shui is the idea of position. When choosing a site on which to settle, the ancient Chinese studied the landscape for sacred symbols, represented by the presence of water, for example, the shape of a lake, the smell of the rain, the appearance of the leaves on the trees, or the way in which wind rushes through a valley. Feng shui experts have adapted this concept to the modern landscape, both urban and rural. They also incorporate astrology and Taoist principles into the making of their assessment, and use all of their senses—not just touch, taste, smell, sight, and hearing, but also latent ones. With these they pick up atmospheric signs and energy patterns similar to those detected during dowsing (seeking underground water by using a divining rod).

When is feng shui used?
Sometimes feng shui is employed at the design stage of a building to ensure that the location is ideal and that the best construction techniques and layout are used. More often, however, a feng shui master is asked to remedy existing problems. This is particularly true in towns and cities where space is at a premium.

How can feng shui reduce stress?
When you use color, light, plants, textures, and furniture in a way that will promote a feeling of harmony with your surroundings, you create a space that will increase your sense of well-being.

WHAT YOU CAN DO AT HOME

USING FENG SHUI
Use this example of a house's layout, room by room, to help you position furniture and plants in order to obtain the most propitious force for your life.

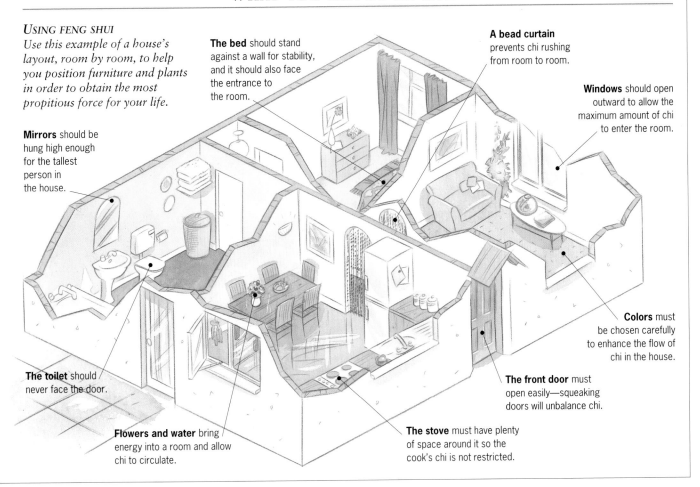

The bed should stand against a wall for stability, and it should also face the entrance to the room.

A bead curtain prevents chi rushing from room to room.

Windows should open outward to allow the maximum amount of chi to enter the room.

Mirrors should be hung high enough for the tallest person in the house.

Colors must be chosen carefully to enhance the flow of chi in the house.

The toilet should never face the door.

The front door must open easily—squeaking doors will unbalance chi.

Flowers and water bring energy into a room and allow chi to circulate.

The stove must have plenty of space around it so the cook's chi is not restricted.

Home Health Spa

Giving yourself the benefits of a relaxing and refreshing spa in your own home is neither difficult nor necessarily expensive. Sometimes the smallest comforts, such as warm towels or sweet-smelling bath oil, can make a world of difference.

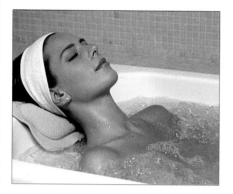

WHIRLPOOL BATHS
The benefits of warm water can be further enhanced by the massage action of water jets, which channel water into a fine or coarse spray. A similar effect can be achieved by spraying a handheld shower against your body.

Water has been used for relaxation and therapy in many different cultures. An essential part of life in ancient Rome was the bathhouse, where Romans went to relax and socialize. You, too, can make your bathroom a refuge, where you can soak away your cares.

Fill your bathtub with water that is just hand hot. This temperature will reduce your heart rate and promote a calming effect. If the water is too warm, your blood vessels will dilate and your heart rate will increase, putting additional physical stress on your body. For extra relaxation, add some essential oils or fragrant herbs to your bath (see page 68). Once you are in the tub, practice deep breathing (see page 39) and visualization (see page 147) and soak for 15 to 20 minutes. Add more hot water to keep the water temperature comfortable.

Follow your soak with a shower, starting with hand-hot water to continue the calming and relaxing effects of your bath. After a few minutes, switch to cooler water, then finish with a brief and invigorating cold shower. This should leave you pleasantly glowing. When you are dry, you will be ready for a massage.

THE POWER OF "NATURAL" BATHING

Many natural products can be used to help ease tired muscles, relieve tension, or invigorate you. You can experiment with oils and salts in your bathwater, or use natural applications directly on your skin.

Soft towels can be used to rub your body down, invigorating and stimulating you after your bath.

To moisturize dry and flaky skin, add 1 to 2 tablespoons heavy cream and a few drops fresh lemon juice to the bathwater.

To exfoliate skin, mix together 1 tablespoon oatmeal and 1 tablespoon honey. Apply to face. Allow to dry before washing off.

BATH ENHANCERS
There are many ways to enhance the revitalizing and relaxing effects of a bath.

Pumice, loofah or exfoliating cream can be used to remove dead skin cells.

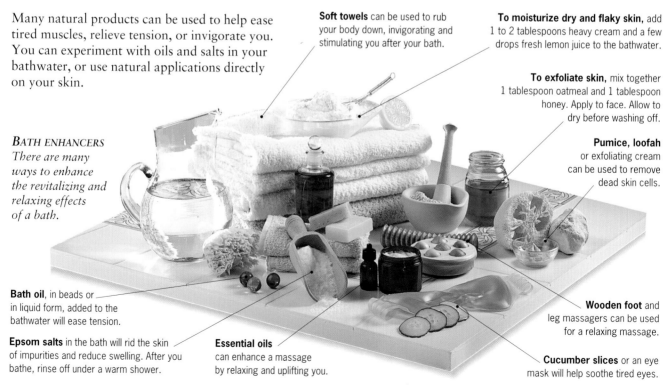

Bath oil, in beads or in liquid form, added to the bathwater will ease tension.

Epsom salts in the bath will rid the skin of impurities and reduce swelling. After you bathe, rinse off under a warm shower.

Essential oils can enhance a massage by relaxing and uplifting you.

Wooden foot and leg massagers can be used for a relaxing massage.

Cucumber slices or an eye mask will help soothe tired eyes.

MASSAGING THE FACE

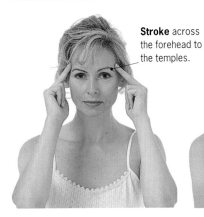

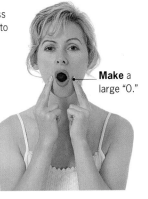

Stroke across the forehead to the temples.

Make a large "O."

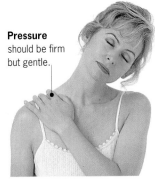

Pressure should be firm but gentle.

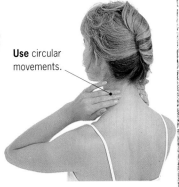

Use circular movements.

FOREHEAD AND TEMPLES
From the center of your forehead, stroke outward to your temples with gentle soothing motions of your fingertips. After a minute or so, press gently on your temples to complete this calming massage.

AROUND THE MOUTH
With your index and middle fingers, make small circular motions over your chin and mouth. Exercise the muscle around your mouth by making a large "O" shape, keeping your lips pressed against your teeth.

NECK AND SHOULDERS
Using your left hand and starting under your ear at the base of your head, stroke down your neck, right shoulder, and right arm. Keep the pressure firm and smooth. Repeat three times, then massage your left side.

BACK OF NECK
Press gently but firmly on the muscle on either side of your spine with the fingertips of both hands. Using circular movements, gently work up your neck to the base of your head and back down again.

MASSAGING THE LEGS

Massaging tired leg muscles will not only relieve aches and tension but also stimulate circulation. Done regularly, it can improve the appearance of your legs as well. You can achieve the best results by completing the whole sequence on one leg before beginning on the other.

STROKE EACH LEG
Working from the ankle to the hip, stroke the leg, as shown at right, pressing firmly and smoothly. Repeat three times.

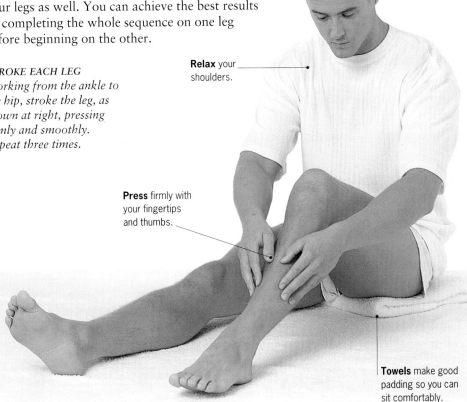

Relax your shoulders.

Press firmly with your fingertips and thumbs.

Towels make good padding so you can sit comfortably.

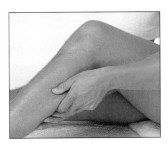

KNEAD THE CALF
Squeeze the muscle away from the bone, then release it. Stroke gently from the ankle to the back of the knee, one hand following the other.

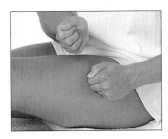

PUMMEL THE THIGH
With loose wrists, work the front and sides of your thigh. This will ease any stiffness in your muscles.

RECIPE FOR A ROOM SPRAY

Choose your favorite fragrance or tailor one to match your mood, and create your own refreshing room spray, using the following recipe:

▶ *10 drops of an essential oil of your choice*

▶ *7 tablespoons of water*

▶ *1 tablespoon of pure alcohol or vodka*

Mix all the ingredients together and pour into a clean spray bottle. The alcohol will help to preserve the essential oil.

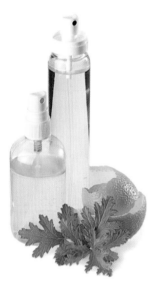

CHOOSING A SCENT
Geranium and orange oils are an effective combination. Geranium is a sedative but it is also uplifting, and may help to ease nervous tension and relieve depression. The scent of oranges adds an energizing note to the blend.

and take a few breaths of fresh air, then go back in and sniff the rooms. Your ability to smell specific things lasts a short while, so try to identify anything unpleasant as soon as you come back inside. You may find that you have become accustomed to an odor that you would now rather do without. Then take steps to eliminate it—for instance, by improving the ventilation, repairing any areas of plaster or wallpaper where mold may have taken hold, repairing damaged drain pipes, or removing a strong-smelling potpourri.

Using essential oils

After eliminating unpleasant smells, you might want to add some pleasing ones to your home. Prepare a room spray, using the recipe at left, pour it into a metal or glass sprayer (a plastic one may degrade), shake well, and spray it around your rooms. You can also place a drop of an essential oil on a cotton ball and set this behind a radiator or inside a heating vent.

Another approach is to release the fragrance of an oil by gently heating it, either in a saucer of water, to which a few drops of the oil have been added, or with a candle. To create an exotic, intimate atmosphere, use sandalwood or patchouli; to unwind in the evening, try geranium or lavender or ylang-ylang. For a lighter touch, orange, lemongrass, or neroli are popular choices. Lavender is often recommended for bedrooms, and will always make your guest room inviting to visitors.

Potpourri, joss sticks, incense, and air fresheners are good alternatives to essential oils. Potpourri that has faded can be revived by adding a few drops of aromatherapy oil. An herbal pillow or scented wooden blocks and paper lining for shelves or drawers can also be pleasing.

PLANTS AND PETS

Houseplants can transform a living space, making it more appealing and attractive. They can add interest to a dull area, divide up spaces, or soften awkward corners. And certain plants have the ability to enhance your environment in more specific ways. The scented leaves of pelargoniums, for example, release a powerful fragrance when their leaves are touched or pressed. The weeping fig (*Ficus benjamina*) is a great general air freshener; Boston fern (*Nephrolepis*

exaltata bostoniensis) is good for removing noxious fumes; and pothos (*Epipremnum aureum*) can remove carbon monoxide.

Even when limited to a terrace or window box, gardening can be very soothing and satisfying. Just seeing the plants that you have tended grow and flourish can provide immeasurable pleasure.

Pets in your household can also enhance it; they are surprisingly effective in reducing stress. Studies have shown that animal owners have less anxiety, lower blood pressure, and generally better health compared with nonowners. Some doctors in Great Britain have been giving out unusual prescriptions to patients suffering from mild depression or stress, or who are recovering from heart attacks: twice-weekly visits to a charitable trust that cares for donkeys and ponies. Just being with the animals and helping with their care has made it possible for these patients to reduce the amount of medication they are taking.

You might not be able to pet fish, but they, too, are excellent reducers of stress. Researchers have found that dental patients who waited in a room with fish swimming in a tank had far less anxiety than those who had no fish to watch. Many institutions for the elderly and the mentally ill have also noted that individuals who keep fish seem to be less lonely and much calmer.

REPAIRS

Allowing household repairs and maintenance chores to pile up can add unnecessary stress to your life. An annoyance such as a squeaking door or dripping faucet may keep you from relaxing at the end of a hard day. Clogged plumbing or a malfunctioning furnace could become a full-blown emergency. To keep on top of things, make a list of all maintenance jobs that must be done regularly, such as changing a filter or cleaning a chimney, and tend to them at the scheduled times. Set aside at least an hour each week for small repairs; you will get instant satisfaction every time you draw a line through a completed task.

For larger problems, such as a leaking roof, make a plan showing how you can save up to have the repair done, when doing the work will be possible, and who will do it. This way you can stop worrying aimlessly, do what needs to be done, and get on with the more enjoyable aspects of your life.

HOME SAFETY

By making sure that your home is accident proof and can't be broken into by burglars, you will be able to reduce considerably your levels of anxiety and stress.

Your home may be a refuge but it also has potential hazards—fire, bodily injury, asphyxiation, and poisoning. Every year, 4 million Americans are injured in home accidents; 27,000 die from them. Here are ways to make your home safer.

You can greatly reduce the risks of fire and electric shock by taking note of possible dangers, such as articles left near an open flame, a carelessly extinguished cigarette stub, or the fraying cord on an electrical appliance. A sensible measure is to have

MAKING THE HOME SAFE FOR THE ELDERLY

A decline in their agility can leave elderly people particularly vulnerable to household accidents. The bathroom, kitchen, and stairs are the most hazardous places, but with a little care all areas in the home can be made much safer.

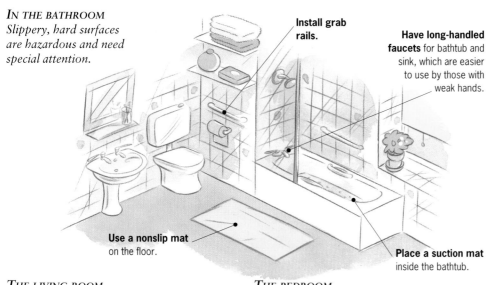

IN THE BATHROOM
Slippery, hard surfaces are hazardous and need special attention.

Install grab rails.

Have long-handled faucets for bathtub and sink, which are easier to use by those with weak hands.

Use a nonslip mat on the floor.

Place a suction mat inside the bathtub.

THE LIVING ROOM
Keep the area free of clutter, such as electrical cords and small rugs, which may cause falls.

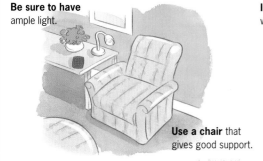

Be sure to have ample light.

Use a chair that gives good support.

THE BEDROOM
Provide for the possibility of having to get out of bed during the night.

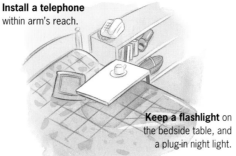

Install a telephone within arm's reach.

Keep a flashlight on the bedside table, and a plug-in night light.

smoke alarms installed on each floor of your home, and change their batteries regularly (usually about twice a year). Make sure that there are at least two possible ways to escape in an emergency. If the house has more than one story, consider keeping a rope ladder upstairs, and have family members practice using it. Buy an all-purpose fire extinguisher and store it in an easily accessible place in or near the kitchen, where most home fires occur.

If you have a gas furnace, make certain that it is properly ventilated, and install a carbon monoxide detector nearby (convenient battery-operated types are available).

Store all medicines, cleaning materials, and toxic chemicals in their original containers, with adequate labeling, and out of the reach of children.

Keep a comprehensive first-aid kit on hand, remember where it is, and bone up now and then on how to use its contents.

CHILDPROOFING THE HOME
By following the suggestions on these pages and ensuring that your children live in the safest environment possible, you will help reduce the worry and stress that can accompany the joys of bringing up a family. Making your home safe for a young child is not difficult or expensive; it simply requires a few precautions, so that natural curiosity and the urge to explore do not put him or her in danger of injury.

CRIME PREVENTION IN THE HOME
While crime of any sort is distressing, the invasion, however slight, of our own "inner sanctum," the one place where we and our loved ones are supposed to be inviolate, has a special power to shock and horrify us. The psychological consequences of a burglary usually far outweigh the material loss. But you can protect your possessions and create a greater sense of security in your home by

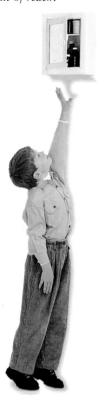

THINGS TO WATCH OUT FOR Medicines should be kept in childproof containers and stored in a cabinet out of reach.

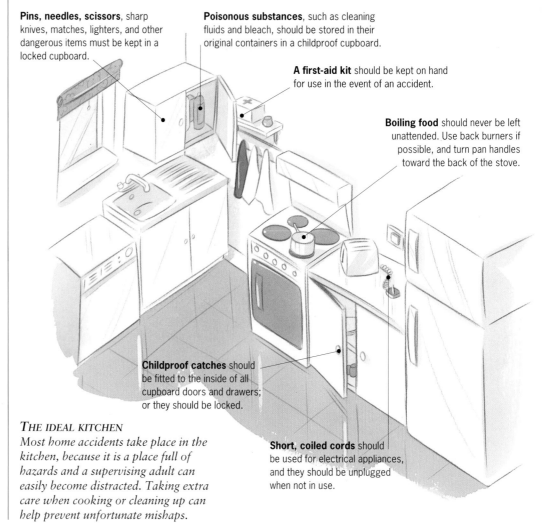

Pins, needles, scissors, sharp knives, matches, lighters, and other dangerous items must be kept in a locked cupboard.

Poisonous substances, such as cleaning fluids and bleach, should be stored in their original containers in a childproof cupboard.

A first-aid kit should be kept on hand for use in the event of an accident.

Boiling food should never be left unattended. Use back burners if possible, and turn pan handles toward the back of the stove.

Childproof catches should be fitted to the inside of all cupboard doors and drawers; or they should be locked.

Short, coiled cords should be used for electrical appliances, and they should be unplugged when not in use.

THE IDEAL KITCHEN Most home accidents take place in the kitchen, because it is a place full of hazards and a supervising adult can easily become distracted. Taking extra care when cooking or cleaning up can help prevent unfortunate mishaps.

taking a surprisingly small number of precautionary measures (see box below). At the same time, you should check your home insurance policy to be sure that it covers your valuables sufficiently, and make an inventory of them, including photographs if possible. If something is stolen, you'll have a good record for the insurance company.

MAKE YOUR HOME YOUR CASTLE

Burglaries and other crimes are not the only threats to privacy and security at home. Many types of intrusion can occur, often without a foot being set in the home or any recognized offense being committed. Such intrusions create their own, often equally disturbing stresses, and it helps to build up defenses against them. For instance, most of us have suffered from telemarketing at inconvenient times or the unwelcome attentions of door-to-door salespersons. Some people have been constantly irritated by neighbors who are insensitive (permitting unreasonable noise from cars, motorcycles, stereos, or dogs); inconsiderate (allowing their weeds and overgrown plants to encroach on others' property, or taking up too much parking space); or just downright unpleasant (taking every opportunity to voice the smallest grievance in the most aggressive manner). The only way to deal with these intrusions effectively is by being assertive (see page 74). When you give a clear, public definition to your personal space, you may avoid some of the disputes that often occur in daily life.

CRIMES IN THE HOME
Although the media provides lots of scare stories, increasing people's fear of burglary, in reality the likelihood of it happening is small. Figures have been coming down in the US, and are still quite low in the UK.

HOME BURGLARY		
YEAR	US*	UK*
1982	7.8%	2.1%
1987	6.2%	2.5%
1992	4.9%	3.7%

*Percentage of households

PREVENTING BREAK-INS

Most burglaries take place during daylight hours. They increase during the summertime, when open doors and windows are an invitation to would-be burglars. The majority of break-ins are not the work of professional criminals but of opportunists taking advantage of someone else's carelessness. Compare this model home with yours to see what you can do to deter casual crime and make your home more burglarproof.

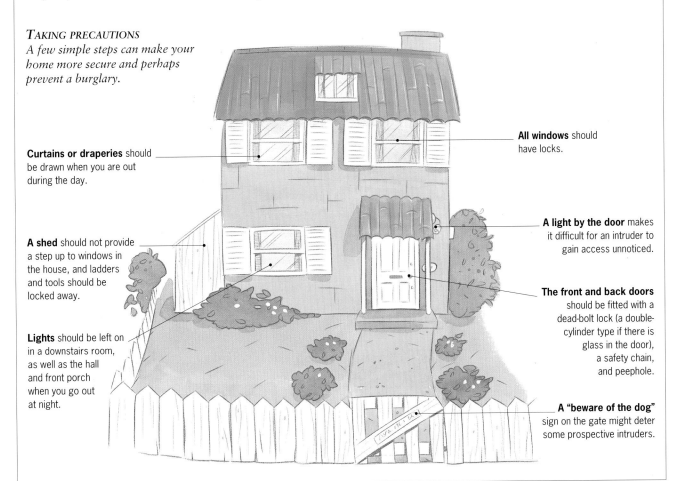

TAKING PRECAUTIONS
A few simple steps can make your home more secure and perhaps prevent a burglary.

Curtains or draperies should be drawn when you are out during the day.

A shed should not provide a step up to windows in the house, and ladders and tools should be locked away.

Lights should be left on in a downstairs room, as well as the hall and front porch when you go out at night.

All windows should have locks.

A light by the door makes it difficult for an intruder to gain access unnoticed.

The front and back doors should be fitted with a dead-bolt lock (a double-cylinder type if there is glass in the door), a safety chain, and peephole.

A "beware of the dog" sign on the gate might deter some prospective intruders.

CELEBRATIONS AND ENTERTAINING

Social get-togethers can be sources of great joy, but hosting them puts extra demands on time, energy, and money. Realistic expectations plus careful planning can help limit the stress.

Human beings are social animals who like to entertain and be entertained by others. But the process is not effortless. A pleasurable event takes thoughtful planning and preparation by the hosts, and consideration on the part of the guests in giving a prompt answer to an invitation, arriving on time, taking an active but not domineering part in conversation, and leaving at an appropriate time.

Successful party givers manage to gather a lively blend of guests. A way to do this is to mix people who have interesting things to say with others who are good listeners, and make sure that the company share some interests but not all are in the same line of work (persistent shop talk can make for a very dull event). If a newcomer is included in a group of people who know each other

well, it is considerate to have at least one person there whom the outsider knows or at least has mutual interests with.

If you are reluctant to entertain because of limited time and/or money, consider sharing the hosting duties with friends. Have dinner at one house, and dessert and coffee at another. Or you might want to go in together on the cost of having an event catered, or of taking mutual friends out.

When you see a sale for a roast or some other food that you would serve for dinner guests, buy it and put it in the freezer for your next party. Do the same for specials at a wine store. You always save money by preparing food yourself, but if your time is very limited, it might be better to spend more and include some take-out food in the menu. For whatever you cook, select recipes that you can prepare ahead of time, saving the hassle of last-minute preparations.

FAMILY GET-TOGETHERS

Graduation parties and wedding showers, Thanksgiving and Mother's Day, these are among the special occasions that afford opportunities to be with people you feel close to. But there can be pitfalls. Family members will usually want to participate in the planning and preparations. If there are differing views on who should be invited, what food to serve, what music to play, and so on, diplomacy is called for.

When the event is in your home, you have the right to do it largely your way, but you still need to consider others' suggestions, especially if you expect them to help with the preparations. Encouraging everyone to contribute something will usually be more satisfying than having a perfect combination of foods or exquisite decorations. If

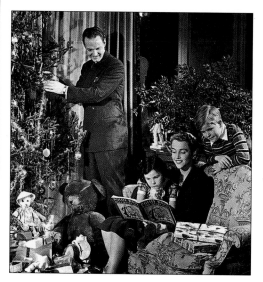

A HAPPY CHRISTMAS?
Christmas is usually a time of family togetherness, but holiday preparations and expectations often put extra stress on relationships.

any members of your family are feuding, or if there is a relative who often creates confusion or irritates others, you might assign special tasks at the party that will keep them too busy to cause tension. You could perhaps allay your fears by speaking to them ahead of time about your concerns. You may find that they are willing, for the sake of the occasion, to modify their behavior or perhaps even bury the hatchet.

CHILDREN'S PARTIES

Children's parties present special challenges, but they can be the most rewarding events. As a rule, it is best to limit the number of guests to a few close friends, especially if you live in an apartment. However, if your child wants to invite a larger group, consider renting a hall in a church, community center, or day-care facility, or using a nearby park, and hire a couple of teenagers or ask another parent or two to help out.

Appropriate activities are the keys to a successful party. For preschoolers, simple games such as Pin the Tail on the Donkey, or a treasure hunt for small candies or favors are fine. Elementary school children usually enjoy memory and guessing games.

This is also a good age for an outing to a zoo, ice skating rink, or movie.

When planning a party for teenagers, set firm rules about attendance (invited guests only), alcohol (none will be allowed), and music (decibel levels will be limited). It's probably a good idea to notify neighbors of the coming event and tell them what time the party will be over. Be sure to have plenty of food and soft drinks on hand and, if you can, provide some activity, such as ping-pong. Also, plan to be at home. You can help greet the young people, then retire to another part of the house.

PARTY PLANNING

Be realistic about how long preparations will take. Experience, of course, is the best guide, but if you are planning a large event of a sort you've never done before, consult a friend who has, or consider using a party planner. You may be surprised at how far ahead you must start (see box, page 116).

Break down tasks into manageable units. Consider offers of help, but accept them only from those who can be relied on to do what they promise. Be clear about what you want, how you want it done, and by when.

Passive smoke

Nowadays, an increasing number of people have never smoked or have stopped, and those who continue to do so find that their habit is far less acceptable than it once was. In fact, just as fewer public places allow smoking, many households have banned it altogether.

If you are having a party and you know that a few guests are smokers, you don't have to allow them to pollute your home. However, you don't want to make them feel unwelcome either. A sensible compromise is to tell guests beforehand that you don't allow smoking in your home, and then give them somewhere relatively warm and dry where they can smoke if they want to, such as a garage or glassed-in porch with plenty of ventilation.

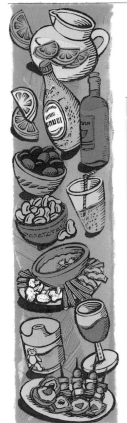

STRESS-FREE ENTERTAINING

Some hosts and hostesses are so busy and stressed that they have little time to spend with guests or enjoy the party. These tips may help to make your next social event fun for everyone.

TIPS FOR A SUCCESSFUL PARTY

▶ *Select a theme for an event. Telling guests that you are planning an Italian dinner or come-as-you-are brunch sets a mood of anticipation.*

▶ *Keep things simple. The goal should be to put guests at ease and for them to have fun, rather than impressing them with elaborate food and decorations.*

▶ *Allow yourself plenty of time for preparations, so that you are calm when guests arrive. Make a list of everything to be done, see if you can delegate any tasks, and prepare as much as possible in advance.*

▶ *If you are serving alcohol, be sure to offer a selection of non-alcoholic beverages as well.*

▶ *Try to remember what you forgot the last time you held a social gathering, and check that you have remembered it this time.*

▶ *Steer guests clear of topics that you know they might strongly disagree upon. Political discussions may be okay for some gatherings but not for others.*

▶ *Feel free to serve some ready-made foods. Today, people accept the fact that those who lead busy lives don't have time to prepare every meal from scratch.*

▶ *Serve dishes that you have made and enjoyed before. There is nothing more stressful than trying to cope with a disappointing or failed recipe in front of company.*

A drink or two

Social gatherings often include alcohol, but today many people do not drink. Below are two festive fruit punches, to which you can add alcohol if you choose, or you can serve them as nonalcoholic alternatives.

RASPBERRY FRUIT PUNCH
Mix together in a large bowl 8 ounces raspberry fruit purée, 3 cups pineapple juice, 2 cups fresh orange juice, 3 tablespoons fresh lemon juice, and 1 tablespoon sugar. If you like, add 2 cups rum.

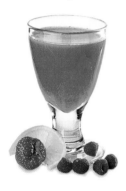

CITRUS FRUIT PUNCH
Bring to a boil 8 cups water, 1½ cups sugar, 1 teaspoon each ground ginger and cinnamon; cook for 5 minutes. Add 2 cups fresh orange juice and 1 cup grapefruit juice; stir well. Add 2 cups gin if you like. Decorate with mint and fruit.

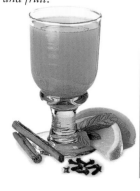

How far ahead should you invite guests? If people must make travel plans, three to six months is not too much notice, but the formal invitation may go out six weeks in advance. For a Saturday-night dinner, three weeks' notice is usually sufficient. Many people don't mind being invited at the last moment for casual come-as-you-are events. Sometimes these are the most fun.

Include time in your plans for relaxation before the party begins. You might listen to favorite music, have a soak in the bath, or just spend 15 minutes with your feet up. Or you may want to break away completely, perhaps by going for a walk. Include it in your schedule though, or you may be working on preparations even as guests arrive.

Once the party is under way, concentrate on making the company feel at home rather than fussing with details, and bear in mind that you and your family are responsible for guests for only a few hours, not a lifetime.

A 50TH WEDDING ANNIVERSARY

George and Martha Brown will be celebrating 50 years of marriage six months from now. Their daughter, Elizabeth, wants to give a big party for family, friends, former colleagues, and neighbors. Because she lives in a small apartment, she has decided the party should be held in the basement of the church where her parents are members. Elizabeth and her son, Paul, live some distance from her parents' home, so many of the arrangements will have to be done with the help of others.

THREE MONTHS BEFORE

Make a preliminary booking for the church.

Investigate hotels and motels in the area where the out-of-town relatives can stay.

Ask parents for names for invitation list. Buy or make invitations and send them out. Ask people to arrange their own hotel reservations; enclose a list of places.

Make reservations for herself and Paul to fly to her parents' home two days before the celebration.

TWO MONTHS BEFORE

Contact Suzanne (an old friend in her hometown) for help. Ask her to gather together some tapes of music reminiscent of the time when Elizabeth's parents got married.

Order the cake, deciding with the store on the type, what is to be written on it, the size, and the price. Send a deposit.

Contact one of the women at the church about organizing a few others to make coffee and punch and to serve drinks and the cake. Find out if they can provide a punch bowl, coffeemaker, and sound system. Offer to make a donation to the church fund.

ONE MONTH BEFORE

Hire a photographer to take pictures.

Arrange for her parents' wedding photograph to be blown up, for use as part of the decorations. Order flowers and special anniversary napkins.

Write lists of the things to buy and do when she arrives in her hometown.

Decide what she and Paul are going to wear.

Contact a relative or close family friend and ask him or her to make a speech at the party.

TWO DAYS BEFORE

Fly to her parents' town.

Contact the church organizer and her friends to make sure that all the arrangements have been carried out.

Arrange for the cake to be delivered to the church.

Visit the church to check out the hall.

Buy decorations for the church hall, and glasses, cups, plates, and cuttlery for the refreshments.

ONE DAY BEFORE

Buy a variety of snack foods and beverages for the party.

Spend the afternoon calling hotels and motels in the area to make sure that all the relatives have arrived safely and that they have organized a way of getting to the church.

Arrange for one of the relatives to take her parents to the church.

Write out the place cards for the guests.

Arrange for the flowers to be delivered to the church.

THE MORNING OF THE CELEBRATION

Get up early and check list of things to do.

Go to the church, put up decorations, and set up the music system.

Pay for the cake and flowers on delivery and make sure that the tables are set up as planned.

Decorate the tables and set out food and beverages.

Leave enough time for a relaxing bath before changing into party clothes.

Celebrate!

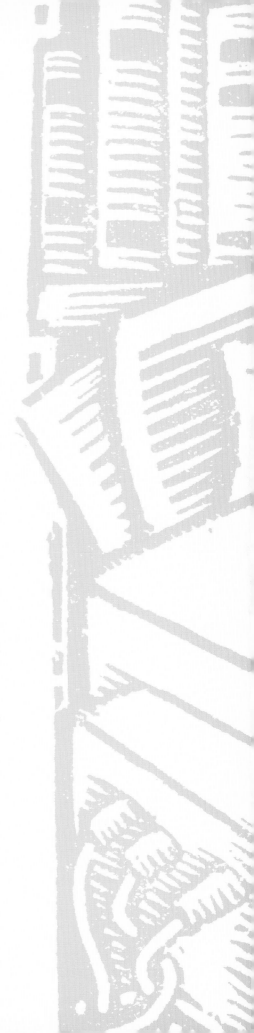

CHAPTER 7

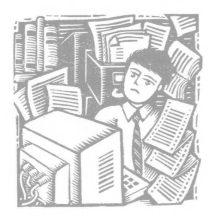

STRESS AT WORK

People under a great deal of stress at work are more likely to suffer injuries and poor mental and physical health. For companies, the consequences of this are absenteeism, high staff turnover, and reduced productivity. Some firms have set up wellness programs to teach employees how to stay healthy and reduce stress through diet, exercise, and relaxation. In this chapter you'll learn how to spot the signs of job stress and discover ways to cope with it effectively.

IS YOUR JOB MAKING YOU STRESSED?

Job stress is America's leading adult health problem. There are many ways to cut down on job stress. A good way to start is to choose a job that matches your personality and your job.

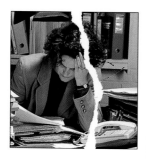

ARE YOU UNDER STRESS? *Work can induce high levels of tension in even the most easygoing people. It can also create stress-related health problems, such as headaches and stomach disorders. There are steps you can take to make even the worst jobs more pleasurable.*

In the wake of increasing competition, downsizing, and bigger demands on individual performance, workers everywhere are experiencing rising levels of job stress. The toll on industry is heavy; it costs thousands of dollars in absenteeism, lost productivity, and work-related accidents each year. Worker's compensation awards for job stress have risen exponentially in the last decade. In California alone, job claims rose 531 percent between 1980 and 1986.

Job stress is not confined to managers and executives. In fact, it affects workers at all levels regardless of their job title or amount of responsibility. In a recently completed 10-year study of British civil servants, researchers found that men and women in the lowest positions, who worked for overbearing and difficult bosses, were three times more likely to become ill than similarly employed workers who had some degree of authority or control over their jobs.

While job stress is difficult to define, at its essence is the bearing of responsibility accompanied by little authority. It's important to remember, however, that what is an unbearable stress to one worker may be an exciting challenge to another. While some people thrive in a hectic work environment, others feel overwhelmed. Much depends on the worker's personality. In fact, most cases of job stress could be avoided if a person's characteristics were more appropriately matched to their job. For instance, putting an energetic go-getter in assembly-line work will soon lead to job stress, as will placing a quiet, unassuming person in the role of spokesperson for a high-profile company.

TOP 10 CAUSES OF STRESS AT WORK

In a May 1984 study by *International Management* of over 1,000 executives in five countries, work pressures were ranked on a scale of 1 to 10, with 1 as the most stressful. Time pressures and work overload were the most highly rated.

STRESSORS	US	UK	GERMANY	SWEDEN	JAPAN
Time pressures and deadlines	2	1	1	2	1
Work overload	1	3	2	1	2
Too much travel	8	2	7	6	7
Long hours	4	4	3	3	5
Taking work home	6	7	8	4	9
Lack of power and influence	3	6	5	10	8
Keeping up with technology	10	5	10	7	3
Inadequately trained subordinates	7	9	4	5	6
Bad interpersonal relations	9	8	9	8	4
Incompetent boss	5	10	6	9	10

Here are some of the major elements of job stress: inadequate time to complete a job, lack of control or pride over one's work, little recognition or reward for a job well done, unpleasant working conditions, such as noise or overcrowding, not being able to use one's abilities, and a lack of clear objectives or support from management.

Other aspects of job stress have to do with the hours and logistics of the job, such as excessive shift work, long hours, extended periods of monotonous or repetitive tasks, constant change in work patterns, too much work-related travel, unrealistic deadlines, and having too much or too little to do.

Job stress typically results from a combination of circumstances that are unique in each industry. A study at an American automobile factory, for instance, identified four key factors that led to job stress: a heavy workload, restrictive company rules, conflicts with colleagues and superiors, and having no control or influence on the work being carried out. What appears to upset workers most is the loss of dignity and pride resulting from management's indifference to workers' comfort and satisfaction.

Other frustrations and anxieties are connected to job insecurity. Rumors of layoffs cause job stress, as does talk of one's company transferring employees to another part

Pathway to health

A few simple tips can help make your workday a little more pleasant. If you are desk-bound most of the time, remember to do stretching exercises every hour or so. A five-minute walk around the office every few hours will refresh you for your next task.

Find an aerobic exercise class to attend at lunchtime or right after work. Far from being tiring, such exercise is more likely to invigorate you and relieve mental stress.

Keep your food intake constant from day to day. A regular breakfast and lunch will stop you from feeling lethargic in the afternoon, while skipping breakfast or eating a large lunch will reduce energy levels.

Keep a bottle of mineral water nearby; drinking water will reduce your intake of coffee and tea, which can overstimulate the nervous system.

Do not take your troubles home with you. When you have finished work, try to switch gears. Read a novel on the train ride home or take a route home that will make you feel relaxed. Then enjoy your leisure time.

Perfume for the mind
To stimulate mental alertness, add a few drops of rosemary, basil, or peppermint essential oil to a damp cotton ball. Place the cotton ball in a saucer or container near a radiator or a patch of sunlight or under your desk lamp—the heat will release the oil's aroma.

MASSAGE IN THE WORKPLACE

Massage is one of the best forms of stress relief, and workers in high-stress jobs are increasingly using it as a way to relieve tensions induced by the pressures of their work. Some Wall Street traders now employ massage therapists who give them neck and shoulder massages at their desks. Take a leaf from their book and use the simple techniques below to relax you and recharge your batteries at work.

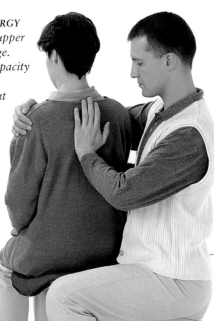

FOR RENEWED ENERGY
Straightening your upper back lifts the rib cage. This expands the capacity of your lungs and increases the amount of oxygen in your bloodstream.

A massage therapist will apply pressure to your back to help release tension in your spine.

FOR RELAXATION
To help ward off rounded shoulders caused by long working hours at a desk, try a regular neck and shoulder massage. It will also give you a feeling of well-being that will last all day.

Firm, consistent pressure will be applied to taut shoulder muscles by a therapist.

HIGH-, MEDIUM-, AND LOW-STRESS JOBS

Using a 10-point scale, psychologists at the University of Manchester in England carried out an assessment of the degree of stress inherent in a range of occupations.

High stress

Miners	*8.3*
Police officers	*7.7*
Construction workers	*7.5*
Airline pilots	*7.5*
Prison wardens	*7.5*
Journalists	*7.5*
Advertising executives	*7.3*
Dentists	*7.3*
Actors	*7.2*
Broadcasters	*6.8*
Firefighters	*6.3*
Ambulance personnel	*6.3*
Personnel officers	*6.0*
Social workers	*6.0*
Public relations officers	*5.8*
Lawyers	*5.7*
Military personnel	*4.8*
Secretaries	*4.7*

Medium stress

Photographers	*4.6*
Pharmacists	*4.5*
Veterinarians	*4.5*
Market researchers	*4.3*
Hairdressers	*4.3*
Accountants	*4.3*
Physiotherapists	*4.2*
Opticians	*4.0*
Architects	*4.0*

Low stress

Computer programmers	*3.8*
Laboratory technicians	*3.8*
Beauty therapists	*3.5*
Church personnel	*3.5*
Bank tellers	*3.3*
Nursery school teachers	*3.3*
Biologists	*3.0*

of the country. Sexual harassment and age discrimination cause a great deal of job stress—a fact that judges and worker's compensation boards consider when determining monetary awards.

Stress and different occupations

Stress is very much an individual concept. Some people might describe a demanding job as "exciting" and "stimulating," while others would call it "exhausting" or "draining." Researchers have found, however, that certain occupations involve a more or less consistent level of pressure, and they are able to group all occupations under the broad categories of high, medium, and low risk (see left). Within these categories, however, both the individual's response to the job and the actual working conditions will influence personal stress levels. Some people whose jobs call for them to face physical danger for which they have been trained and equipped, for example, may in fact have lower stress levels than others who are in relatively safe occupations.

Other jobs may have certain built-in stresses, such as unpleasant confrontations with the public, but have other pleasant aspects that can help to offset these problems. Hairdressers, for example, deal with people all the time, but the job that they are doing is creative and involves touch, two factors that help to counteract stress. Certain occupations, such as that of a market researcher, computer programmer, or bank teller, consist of routine work, which may be quite skilled but does not involve a lot of decision making. These types of jobs, too, are less stress inducing.

Occupations that usually involve well-established routines and little responsibility, such as factory work, however, are often boring and poorly paid, and provide few real challenges. This lack of pressure may suit those who have a low threshold for stress, or have no interest in establishing a career. To a more ambitious person, such a job may cause intense frustration, and he or she will have to move on quickly to another job to avoid the stress of repetitive work.

Combating stress at work

Although it is now universally acknowledged that businesses suffer when their employees are under stress, many companies are still reluctant to deal with the problem. This means that people in the workforce, including the growing number of self-employed, must pay serious attention to their own symptoms of too much stress,

WHAT IS THE POTENTIAL STRESS RATING OF YOUR JOB?

Even a good salary and job satisfaction may involve some work pressures that can affect your health. To find out your level of job stress, think back over the past three months and check all the questions that apply to you. Add up the points. If you have more than eight points, then you are clearly under pressure at work. If the stress is more than you can handle, you should consider getting a different job or making changes to the one you have, to alleviate some of the stress.

QUESTIONS	SCORE
Is your job poorly paid or insecure?	1
Do you have to work in unpleasant conditions?	1
Are you responsible for the mistakes of others?	1
Are you responsible for your own mistakes?	2
Are the consequences of any errors you make likely to cause financial loss or danger to others?	2
Are you solely responsible for your own workload?	2
Do you have strict deadlines or sales targets to meet?	3
Do you have to work long hours to cope with your workload?	3
Do you have to face arguments or confrontations?	3
Do you have to face dangerous situations?	4
TOTAL	

THE POTENTIAL STRESS IN DIFFERENT OCCUPATIONS

The amount of anxiety you feel in a particular occupation depends not only on the stresses inherent in the work but also on you as an individual. Jobs can be of low, medium, or high stress (see opposite page) or only stressful at certain times. Some people would characterize a particular job as pressured or exacting, while others would see the same position as challenging and rewarding. Below are descriptions of six different occupations, together with some of the reasons that they are potentially stressful as well as the ways in which they offer satisfaction.

PHYSICIAN

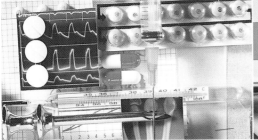

Although this is a respected and generally well-paid profession, the hours can be long and there can be unrealistic demands on the individual. Responsibility for people's lives plus the risk of malpractice suits make the job very stressful.

TEACHER

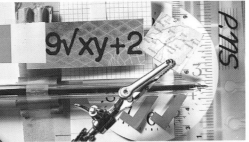

A potentially rewarding job, teaching has a high degree of control. However, the level of stress can be very high if one is not supported by superiors, if the students are not motivated, or if there is a lack of resources.

SELF-EMPLOYED WORKER

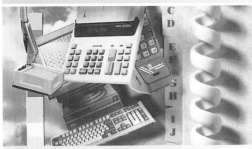

As long as there is plenty of suitableand enjoyable work available, being your own boss can be rewarding. Stress increases when work is scarce and there is a lack of contact with colleagues, which can give rise to feelings of loneliness.

SENIOR EXECUTIVE

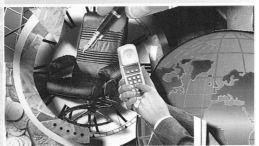

Job satisfaction and benefits are high. Working at this level involves taking responsibility for many others, but there is scope for delegating. Stress arises from long work hours, sometimes a great deal of traveling, and knowing that mistakes can be costly.

OFFICE MANAGER

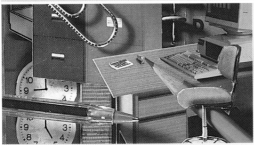

Taking responsibility for work done by others can be stressful—poor performance by a subordinate reflects badly on you. But you will have some control over your work conditions, and you can delegate a few tasks that you dislike.

SALES CLERK

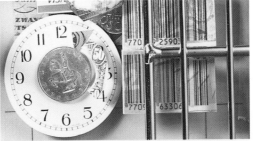

Selling merchandise is sometimes boring and poorly paid, but it is relatively undemanding and carries little responsibility. Dealing with the public can be both pleasurable and stressful, but major problems can normally be passed on to a supervisor.

Dentists' dilemma
A study published in the *Journal of Ocupational Psychology* in 1978 found that American dentists suffer from high levels of stress. The dentists attribute their high stress levels to the conflict caused by their perceptions of them-selves as fulfilling a caring role, and the public's perception of dentists as "inflictors of pain."

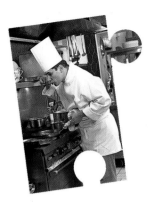

PUTTING IT ALL TOGETHER
Consider all aspects of your personality, as well as practical matters, when choosing a career, and you will lessen your chances of experiencing job frustration.

namely sleeplessness, headaches, stomach problems, or excessive irritability, and develop their own strategies for coping.

The first step to stress reduction is to determine what is really bothering you. Be specific. Vague statements such as "I hate my job," are not helpful. Analyze what it is about the job that is making you unhappy. One common cause of anxiety at work, for example, is not knowing exactly what is expected of you. If this is true in your case, you might ask your boss or personnel manager for written guidelines and schedules. If the problem is a personality conflict with another worker, try to resolve the difficulty with the help of the personnel department or a senior staff member. You might even consider a heart-to-heart with the individual involved. Serious worries should always be referred to a more senior member of the staff or to your union leader.

Changing jobs

You may find that no matter what you do—talking to your boss, coming up with plans to reduce stressful working practices, sorting out differences with colleagues—you are still unhappy and tense at work. In such a case, the only answer is to find another, different type of job, one that has the potential

TAKING STOCK OF YOUR ABILITIES

Employment consultants conduct interviews and tests to find out what type of work will suit their clients, but you can create your own personal profile. The self-knowledge you will gain may give you an idea of where you would best fit in, or explain why you are not happy in your present job. You can also use the information to construct a résumé or to prepare for job interviews or assessments by a consultant. The list below may help you to project your talents, qualifications, leanings, and interests in the best possible light. Read it through, and then write down on a separate piece of paper the statements that apply to each section.

APTITUDES

► Verbal: includes the ability to express yourself and to persuade others, and to read carefully and write clearly.

► Numerical: ability to calculate with figures and formulas, to understand statistics, and to present them clearly.

► Conceptual: includes the ability to construct and follow an argument, and to determine the relationships and sequences within a variety of data.

► Practical: level of manual dexterity; ability to plan in two dimensions and to visualize in three dimensions.

► Creative ability: aptitude for innovation and problem solving; ability to arrive at new ideas and concepts; in some jobs, good artistic and design sense.

► Organizational skills: ability to create order, both mentally and practically; reliability in following tasks through to completion.

► Interpersonal skills: ability to coordinate with, listen to, and influence others.

INTERESTS

► Activities that you currently engage in.

► Activities you would like to pursue.

► Consider how they reflect your personality, and how they relate to and complement your work.

PERSONALITY

Establish your personality type by deciding where you fit between each of these extremes:

► Are you sociable or self-contained?

► Are you excitable or unemotional?

► Are you a leader or a follower?

► Are you rigid or flexible?

► Are you tough-minded or sensitive?

► Are you conforming or independent?

QUALIFICATIONS

► Academic qualifications: examinations, degrees, training courses.

► Professional attainments: range of tasks you have undertaken, depth of experience gained in each, achievements at work.

ASSESSMENT

Look at what you have written and try to find a single thread that runs through it. You need to see the big picture before you can draw conclusions and limit your job choice and field. For instance, if you find that you describe yourself as independent, methodical, and good with numbers, a career in accounting, or perhaps laboratory work or another scientific endeavor might be worth considering.

to provide fulfillment and stimulation. In today's economic climate, however, it would be unwise to remove yourself from one set of problems only to subject yourself to other stresses, namely, financial insecurity. So make your decision to leave but, if possible secure your next job before you say good-bye to what you have.

To find out whether your work is suited to your background and abilities, first complete the questionnaire on the opposite page.

Once you have done this, think about what you want from a job. There are a number of questions to consider. Could you work at a desk job or do you need to get out and meet people? How much travel are you willing to do? Do you desire a job that has a path to promotion? How do you feel about responsibility? Must you have complete control over your work, for example, managing projects from start to finish? Do you want a job that calls for managing people? Are you comfortable delegating tasks? Do you like to work alone or do you want to be part of a team? Do you enjoy working with the public? Does job satisfaction mean more to you than financial reward? How hard are you willing to work?

Also, think about the package you would like. Most companies offer more than just a salary For example, pension and health insurance as well as tuition reimbursement come with many jobs. Consider the type of office environment you would feel most comfortable in and the amount of time you are able to spend commuting to and from work. Also, think about how much overtime you would be willing to put in.

DRESS THE PART FOR YOUR JOB INTERVIEW

First impressions are crucial, so make sure you are appropriately dressed. If you can, spend five minutes outside your prospective workplace the day before your interview and observe the people who work there. You will quickly get an idea of the right clothes to wear.

Hair should be short, or swept up.

FINANCE
Somber colors and conservative styles are essential.

Neckline needs to be high and unfussy.

PUBLISHING
An informal, relaxed style of dressing is acceptable; good grooming will ensure you are taken seriously.

Scarves and jewelry for women will have a softening effect on businesslike attire.

Long hair is acceptable but a good cut is critical.

SALES
Crisp, bright colors are good for making you look approachable, but styles should be classic.

INTERVIEW SUCCESS

Good preparation gives you confidence, thereby reducing anxiety. Keep the following in mind:

▶ *Read the job description carefully. If there is not enough information, phone the company and ask if further details are available.*

▶ *Find out about the company. Check the financial press or any relevant trade journals. If possible, speak to someone who works (or has worked) there. Secure a company brochure or a catalog of their products.*

▶ *Prepare a list of questions in anticipation of being asked "Do you have any questions about the job or the company?"*

▶ *Try visualizing the interview (see page 135) the week before it happens. Run through the entire procedure, from the moment you arrive at the company to when you leave.*

▶ *Look the part. Self-expression through clothing is fine, but if you want the job, dress appropriately (see left).*

▶ *Arrive on time!*

▶ *Take along a copy of your résumé (in case the original has been mislaid) and, if relevant, samples of your work.*

▶ *You are likely to be asked "So, why do you think you're suitable for the job?" Be ready with an answer in terms of work experience, education, relevant interests, and special strengths.*

Body Language

The way you move—or do not move—can reveal a lot about you. If you learn to use gestures and posture to your advantage, it will boost your confidence and help you cope more effectively with stressful situations, both at home and at work.

STRESS-FREE SITUATIONS

The following tips will help you successfully negotiate any stressful situation.

▶ *Visualize anxiety-producing events in advance so that you can desensitize yourself to them (see page 135).*

▶ *If you have something important to say, practice it in private first.*

▶ *Breathe deeply and evenly before a particularly stressful encounter.*

▶ *Think positively—negative thoughts will affect the way you speak and hold yourself.*

Most of us use our bodies as aids in communication—just try talking without making any facial expressions or moving your hands. Body language is a powerful method of communicating, and people often make judgments about each other based on it, especially on eye contact, smiles, and frowns.

The most revealing gestures are those that we make deliberately.

When you greet someone, you can let your actions "speak" your feelings: a vigorous handshake will tell a person that you are glad to see him.

At interviews you will give a better impression if you walk confidently into the interviewer's office, rather than sidling in. Folding your arms across your stomach is often a defensive gesture, whereas avoiding eye contact indicates a lack of confidence.

USING BODY LANGUAGE

If you are aware of the impact your body language has on others, you can use this to great effect, but first you must become aware of any unconscious gestures and learn to control them. Pay close attention to how you respond when you meet a friend. Notice how you move your hands, hold your head, or use facial expressions. Does your body language match what you are trying to say?

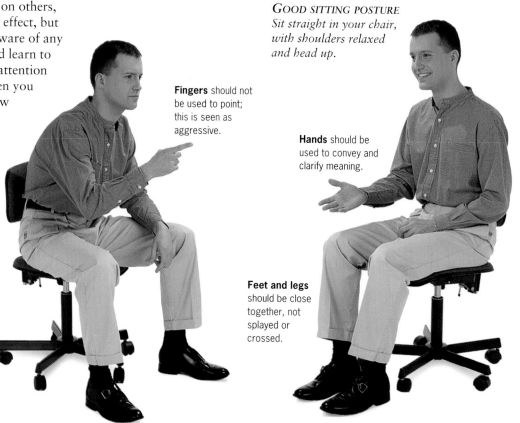

GOOD SITTING POSTURE
Sit straight in your chair, with shoulders relaxed and head up.

Fingers should not be used to point; this is seen as aggressive.

Hands should be used to convey and clarify meaning.

BAD SITTING POSTURE
Slouching gives the impression that you have a negative view of the world.

Feet and legs should be close together, not splayed or crossed.

USING PERSONAL SPACE

How near or far people place themselves in relation to you tells you a great deal about how they feel about you. A person who encroaches inappropriately on another's space is seen as threatening, but if someone you consider a friend withdraws too far, you may feel that he or she no longer likes you or is trying to keep distance between you two for a particular reason.

Tolerable nearness varies with each individual, and is also influenced by cultural factors. If you are from Latin America, the Middle East, or the Mediterranean region, for example, you may feel comfortable within closer limits than someone from northern Europe.

In this crowded world, people often have to move into the space of others, for instance, during a rush-hour bus or train ride or even standing in line at a supermarket checkout or post office. If you are tired, nervous, anxious, or in a hurry, these ordinary situations can become stressful. To make them less so, keep your arms loosely by your side and avoid eye contact. Try to remain relaxed by finding something neutral to focus upon.

HOW CLOSE CAN YOU GET?
Studies have defined four levels of body space that people use in their dealings with others. Each is appropriate for a different level of relationship.

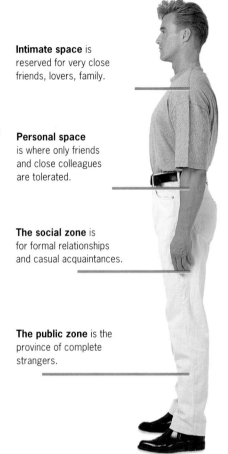

Intimate space is reserved for very close friends, lovers, family.

Personal space is where only friends and close colleagues are tolerated.

The social zone is for formal relationships and casual acquaintances.

The public zone is the province of complete strangers.

READING THE BOSS

To gain important information during meetings, pay attention to the body language of the participants. For example, you may notice your boss touching his or her face a lot. This often demonstrates nervousness. What subjects may be causing this?

When listening to anxiety-provoking subjects, show as much openness as possible. Sit with your legs uncrossed and lean forward a bit. Using relaxed body language when someone else is anxious or aggressive may help to dispel negative feelings.

NEEDS CONVINCING
Her tilted head indicates interest, but strong arguments are needed to win this boss over.

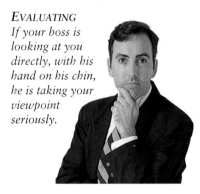

EVALUATING
If your boss is looking at you directly, with his hand on his chin, he is taking your viewpoint seriously.

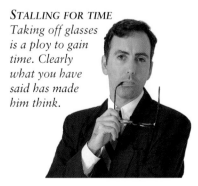

STALLING FOR TIME
Taking off glasses is a ploy to gain time. Clearly what you have said has made him think.

LET YOUR BODY SPEAK FOR YOU

Many people rely on their reading of another person's body language far more than on the words that are spoken to them. For instance, if the body language of a person conflicts with his or her verbal message, that person is less likely to be believed. By following the tips below, you can influence what your own body reveals to others, and use gestures to make positive rather than negative statements.

BODY PART	DO	DON'T
Head	Keep your chin up.	Look at the floor.
Eyes	Make eye-to-eye contact. Use your eyes when you smile.	Hold eye contact for so long that it becomes a stare.
Mouth	Relax the muscles; tension often shows in the mouth.	Smile constantly, clench your teeth, or keep your jaw rigid.
Shoulders	Hold them down and back slightly. Keep them relaxed.	Hunch over—it's a sign of insecurity.
Hands	Use hands for emphasis, but keep gestures small.	Fiddle, play with rings, crack your knuckles—these indicate nervousness.

THE ENVIRONMENT AND THE WORKPLACE

Most of us spend at least half our waking hours at work. No matter the type of workplace—office, factory, or home— we all benefit if it is as healthy and free of stress as possible.

Medical authorities have come to recognize that people do seem to get sick more often while working in some buildings than in others; this phenomenon has been labeled the "sick building syndrome" or SBS.

A World Health Organization committee has estimated that up to 30 percent of new and remodeled buildings may have some air quality problems. A 1992 report from the Health and Safety Executive in Great Britain stated that up to 55 percent of people who worked in air-conditioned buildings in that country could have been adversely affected by poor air quality.

People working in "sick" offices and factories can develop nose and throat irritation, wheezing, headaches, a feeling of lethargy, and eyestrain. Typically, these symptoms appear at work, and are relieved only when the sufferer goes home.

According to the Environmental Protection Agency, SBS is usually caused by three major factors: air pollution from noxious substances, such as cleaning fluids or pesticides; poorly designed ventilation systems; and problems arising from a building being used for purposes for which it was not intended, as when a residential building is used for commercial purposes. Moreover, in an effort to make buildings more energy efficient, architects have made offices and other workplaces sealed units, meaning the heating and air-conditioning systems are out of the employees' control.

To tackle the major causes of SBS, company employees need to present a united front to management, and point out that an unhealthy workforce is much less productive than a healthy one. At the very least, you should ensure that "no smoking" policies are enforced, and that work environments are free of noxious chemicals. Also, ask for environmentally friendly office and factory supplies; they are becoming cheaper and easier to find.

Studies have found that people who work in an office environment where they can see something of nature, such as trees and water, have higher productivity and lower absenteeism than other workers. These findings have brought about changes in design:

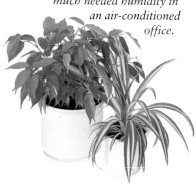

AN OFFICE OASIS
Well-watered plants on your desk can provide much needed humidity in an air-conditioned office.

THE POWER OF PLANTS

NASA scientists working for the US space program have decided that plants are a sure way of cleaning the atmosphere of an enclosed area such as a space station or an office. The human body exhales the waste product carbon dioxide, which can accumulate in poorly ventilated buildings, causing wheezing, breathlessness, and fatigue in people who work there. Plants, however, absorb carbon dioxide, and convert it to oxygen, which is then released into the air, thus making it more breathable.

Plants provide other benefits, too. For instance, just looking at them is refreshing—a reminder of outdoors and a relief from the office environment. But if you need more than a reminder, go out at lunchtime for some fresh air and rest your eyes on some natural greenery.

THE BENEFIT OF IONIZERS

The air you breathe contains electrically charged particles known as ions, mainly created by radiation from the sun and outer space. The ions can be positive or negative, and in the best air they are in equilibrium. But storms and pollution encourage a buildup of positive ions, leaving negative ions in short supply. This imbalance can make people feel unwell. After a storm has passed, people often feel uplifted, due to the return of negative ions in the atmosphere.

IONIZERS
Available as large or small machines, ionizers emit a stream of negative ions, thus improving the balance in the atmosphere.

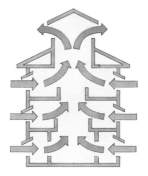

OFFICES THAT BREATHE NATURALLY
Some of today's architects design naturally ventilated structures, in which cool air entering a building is warmed by occupants and equipment and moves toward a central atrium where it is drawn up through a wind tower and expelled.

fountains and waterfalls can often be found in the lobbies and atriums of large new office buildings. Whenever possible, offices should overlook a graceful scene, such as a pond or flower garden. The movement of water will also reduce the amount of pollution in the air.

FENG SHUI IN THE OFFICE
The Chinese art of feng shui makes the best use of the forces of nature by carefully positioning buildings and the objects that are within them in order to promote health, wealth, and happiness, and business success (see page 106).

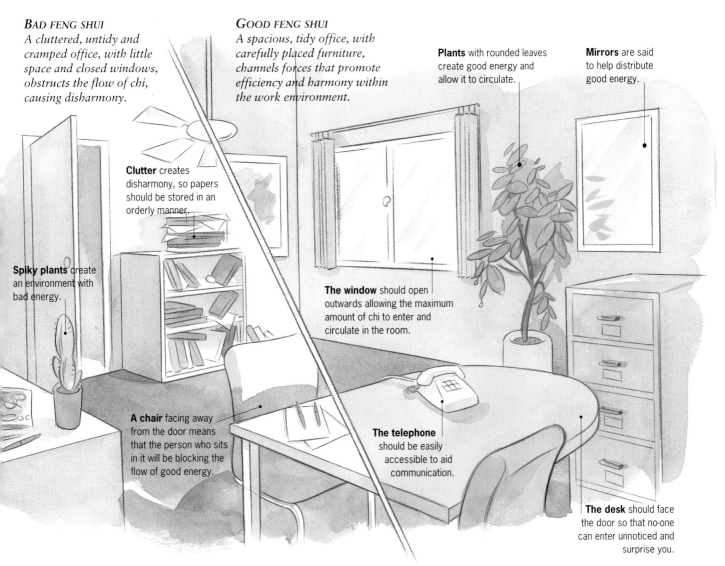

BAD FENG SHUI
A cluttered, untidy and cramped office, with little space and closed windows, obstructs the flow of chi, causing disharmony.

GOOD FENG SHUI
A spacious, tidy office, with carefully placed furniture, channels forces that promote efficiency and harmony within the work environment.

Plants with rounded leaves create good energy and allow it to circulate.

Mirrors are said to help distribute good energy.

Clutter creates disharmony, so papers should be stored in an orderly manner.

Spiky plants create an environment with bad energy.

The window should open outwards allowing the maximum amount of chi to enter and circulate in the room.

A chair facing away from the door means that the person who sits in it will be blocking the flow of good energy.

The telephone should be easily accessible to aid communication.

The desk should face the door so that no-one can enter unnoticed and surprise you.

Keys to success

Networking—making contact with people in a similar field or work situation through professional meetings, social events, and electronic mail—can put you in touch with others in organizations relevant to your work, and also self-employed people who live near you. In addition to the social aspect, you may also find job opportunities or information valuable to your work. Networking can be essential for those who work at home or are in fields where knowledge or technology changes rapidly.

When the Bank of China built a new office in Hong Kong, opposite the Hong Kong and Shanghai Bank, it was believed to have created bad feng shui for all the surrounding firms. A master of the art of feng shui said that the new building's sharp edges acted like daggers, slicing at neighboring buildings. The master ordered many design changes so that good feng shui returned and the bank and its neighbors felt secure.

Masters help to provide good feng shui in workplaces by advising on where particular functions should be carried out, how and where desks should be positioned, and how to block the path of bad feng shui by the judicious placing of objects such as plants, mirrors, and goldfish bowls. The masters claim that a properly sited aquarium with goldfish is an effective way of combating negative influences, but only if there is an odd number of fish in the tank.

A SUCCESSFUL HOME OFFICE

Many people dream of being their own boss, leaving behind office politics and having flexible time for themselves and their families. One way to make that dream come true is to work from your home.

Starting a home office is appealing, especially when you think of all the hours you would save if you no longer had to commute. Other advantages include the freedom of choosing your own working hours (as long as your deadlines are met), and wearing clothes that please you, unconstrained by formal dress codes. While many of these benefits can lead to less stress in your life, working at home can create a whole new set of stresses unless you plan carefully.

To ease yourself into working at home you might consider a situation where you work exclusively for a company or client who provides you with all the necessary equipment, such as a computer, modem, and fax machine. Telemarketing is just one example, but the range of occupations is increasing rapidly.

Problems may arise if, instead of doing a full day's work at home, work takes over all of your home life. It is very easy to lose sight of the importance of free time. With most jobs, when you leave the premises, your time is your own. If your office is in your home, there is nothing to stop you from spending every moment of the day working. Even when you are just starting out, it is important for your health and well-being that you allow a reasonable amount of time for yourself to relax and unwind.

Learning how to schedule your workload is essential. Use a calendar to keep track of when work is coming in, how long you think it will take, when you should make an invoice for it, and when you have received payment. Keep careful records. A paper trail of a project completed on time can be a template for the next one. It will also come in handy when you file your taxes.

THE PROS AND CONS OF STARTING A HOME OFFICE

There are many factors to consider when you contemplate working from home. In addition to the listed advantages, tax breaks may be possible. It is a good idea, therefore, to consult an accountant before setting up a business at home.

ADVANTAGES	DISADVANTAGES
▶ *The sense of liberation that comes from being your own boss.*	▶ *You can feel isolated from the world.*
▶ *If you have a variety of clients, any trouble with some may be outweighed by good relationships with others.*	▶ *A lack of contact with people in your field can lead to worries of being out of touch and left behind.*
▶ *The extra flexibility means you can work when you want, and run the odd errand when it suits you. Child care is made easier, and illnesses cause fewer problems.*	▶ *Family and friends can prevent you getting work done, unless you set clear limits.*
▶ *If it is your own concern, it will be satisfying to know that your hard work results directly in cash in your own pocket.*	▶ *Without a commute to create a separation between your work life and your personal life, you may find it hard to settle down to work.*
▶ *Not having to commute to work.*	▶ *Work can dry up for no reason, and clients can be slow in paying or default altogether.*
	▶ *Many self-employed people take on too much work, and exhaustion can result.*

Also, because there are a number of tax issues involved when starting a home office, you should consult an accountant or lawyer. And don't overlook such essentials as medical insurance and a pension plan.

To help you prioritize your work, use time management strategies (see page 133), and have a clear idea of what tasks need to be tackled first. It is also important to communicate with your clients. While nobody likes being told of a problem, you should inform clients of significant difficulties and, whenever possible, offer solutions

Despite some negative aspects, there is certainly a future for home-office workers, thanks to advances in modern technology. Advocates have high hopes that the benefits of working away from a central office will come to outweigh possible problems.

The stress-free home office

It is important to create a working environment that is conducive to both your health and productivity. Pay special attention to protecting yourself from the distracting noises of the household. Before you start up your home office, talk with your family about the noise factor, and negotiate with them. For instance, music may be played only after certain hours or far away from your office. However, you may have to recognize that there is nothing at all you can do about certain noises, like a dog barking in your neighbor's yard. Consider buying a fan or a machine that makes white noise (see page 143). Locating your home office in a basement or attic may be the answer. Or, if you live in a particularly noisy area, you can soundproof the room.

You should also make sure that your office is well stocked with office supplies. You don't want to have to run out for paper or staples in the middle of an important project—this is not cost effective.

Another skill you will need to acquire is the art of saying no. Family and neighbors will make demands on you once they know you are at home; you will have to be clear about how flexible you can be because, after all, you are working. If you do not set limits early on, you will find yourself getting stressed at yet another interruption.

(see page 133)

WELL-BEING FOR HOME-OFFICE WORKERS

For those who work at home, it is all too easy to remain with your nose to the grindstone hour after hour. Therefore, if you want to remain sane and healthy, you should make a conscious effort to take a 15-minute coffee or tea break every morning and afternoon and eat a nutritionally balanced lunch. If you use a computer, take regular short breaks and do the stretching and flexing exercises shown on the right.

At least once a day, leave the house, if only to mail a letter. You should take this opportunity to move around, getting some fresh air and a change of scenery, as this will refresh you and keep you mentally alert.

When you take your breaks, turn on your answering machine, and once you have finished for the day, close the door to your office, physically and mentally. Although it can be difficult, you should make an effort to separate your work life from your home life.

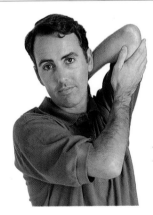

Keep shoulders relaxed throughout.

SHOULDER STRETCH
Lift your left arm, and gently bend it back and down. Repeat with your right arm.

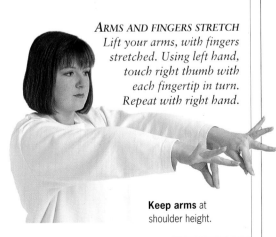

ARMS AND FINGERS STRETCH
Lift your arms, with fingers stretched. Using left hand, touch right thumb with each fingertip in turn. Repeat with right hand.

Keep arms at shoulder height.

BUSINESS PLANS

Business plans are essential if you want to borrow money from a bank to start or expand your business or upgrade your equipment. They will clarify where you are in terms of your career, what you want to do, and how you might go about achieving it. The following are some of the crucial questions you will have to consider when making your business plan.

▶ *What are your products or services?*

▶ *What is your market and what is your place in it?*

▶ *What is the competition like?*

▶ *What progress has your business made over the past three years?*

▶ *How do you see your business developing?*

▶ *What plans have you made to improve or replace your current production or services?*

▶ *What financial goals have you set?*

▶ *What is your financial forecast for next year? For the next five years?*

Computer Work

Many of the physical stresses caused by using a computer, such as back strain, eyestrain, headaches, and upper limb strains, can be avoided or at least minimized by using a properly designed workstation.

CAREFUL LIGHTING

Good lighting in a work area is essential in order to prevent both eyestrain and headaches, and to enable you to work well.

▶ *Windows and lamps should be to one side of the screen only.*

▶ *If glare from sunlight is a problem, fit vertical blinds to the windows (venetian blinds will focus sunlight into pencil-thin beams).*

▶ *Buy special louvers to counteract the glare from light fixtures.*

Millions of people around the world spend most of their working lives at computer terminals. This has resulted in a widespread increase in the range of occupational illnesses, especially repetitive stress injuries or RSI (see opposite page).

These health problems can be prevented if you take a little time and effort. For instance, you will need to assess such things as the height of your workstation and chair, the placement of your computer terminal, and the position and type of your lights. Additionally, correct sitting positions and special exercises may help ward off strain in your hands, arms, and shoulders.

SETTING UP THE IDEAL WORKSTATION

To work efficiently and comfortably, you should be able to make adjustments to your worktable, chair, and computer screen to suit your height, build, weight, and arm positions.

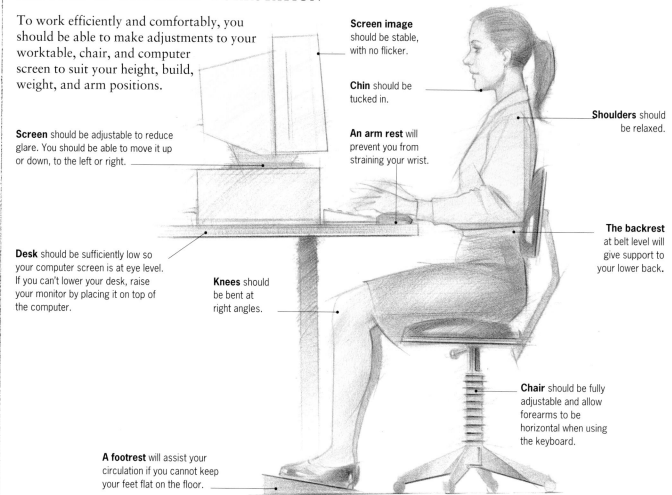

Screen image should be stable, with no flicker.

Chin should be tucked in.

An arm rest will prevent you from straining your wrist.

Shoulders should be relaxed.

Screen should be adjustable to reduce glare. You should be able to move it up or down, to the left or right.

The backrest at belt level will give support to your lower back.

Desk should be sufficiently low so your computer screen is at eye level. If you can't lower your desk, raise your monitor by placing it on top of the computer.

Knees should be bent at right angles.

Chair should be fully adjustable and allow forearms to be horizontal when using the keyboard.

A footrest will assist your circulation if you cannot keep your feet flat on the floor.

PROTECTING YOUR EYESIGHT

Working on a computer does not in itself harm the eyes; however, many people who do intensive work using a computer screen often report having problems with their eyes. Because of this, it makes good sense for anyone who is contemplating or already working on a computer to have his or her eyes examined at regular intervals.

The heat generated by a computer can make the surrounding atmosphere so dry that wearing contact lenses can become difficult for some people. Additionally, computer users tend not to blink as much as other workers, which can also make eyes feel dry. Blinking more often and using eyedrops can help.

Strained eyes can redden, water, or cause headaches. Alleviate such symptoms by exercising your eye muscles. Focus on a spot far away, if possible through a window to the horizon. Next focus on a spot a few feet from you, and then look at something close, like the tip of your nose. Reverse the process, and do the exercise whenever you can. Two more useful eye exercises you can try are illustrated below.

RESTING THE EYES
Cover your closed eyes with your cupped hands for five to 10 minutes, concentrating on pleasant and restful thoughts. Do not let your cupped hands touch your eyes.

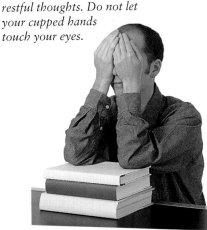

NEAR AND FAR FOCUSING
To exercise the eye muscles, focus on each of two pencils in turn, one six inches from your nose, the other at arm's length. Repeat 10 to 12 times.

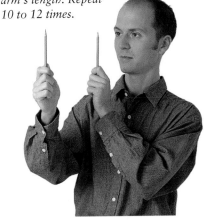

REPETITIVE STRESS INJURY (RSI)

This is an umbrella term that covers various injuries of the hands, arms, and shoulders caused by repeated movements. Some examples are carpal tunnel syndrome (compression of a nerve within the wrist) and tenosynovitis (inflammation of a sheath that covers a tendon).

Repetitive stress injuries can strike anyone who does work that requires excessive hand movement, such as assembly-line workers, musicians, typists, meat packers, and chicken pluckers.

RSI usually starts with a tingling in or numbness of the affected part of the body, or a slight pain that goes away at night but returns when the individual starts to work. If nothing is done, the pain gets worse until it prevents virtually all use of the hand, wrist, arm, or shoulder. This aggravated condition may last for months. If you suspect you have RSI, seek medical treatment immediately.

PLAYING THE VIOLIN
Any activity that involves constant repetitive motions has the capacity to cause RSI.

Learn to relax wrists, neck, and shoulders to prevent RSI.

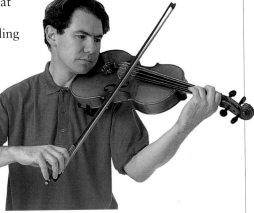

STRESS-BEATERS FOR YOUR MIND AND BODY

Follow these tips to avoid some of the mental and physical strains that commonly arise during work.

▶ *Take regular breaks from your work. Experts recommend taking one every hour, for five to 10 minutes; they believe that frequent, short breaks are better than longer, less frequent ones. If your boss objects to you taking a break, then do a completely different type of work at these times.*

▶ *Avoid holding yourself in static, awkward positions for long periods, and adopt a relaxed position whenever possible. Stretch and flex your hands, arms, shoulders, and neck regularly.*

▶ *Keyboard operators should consider using a padded wrist rest, and look into getting an anti-RSI keyboard (one that is split into two parts so that the hands can be held in less strained positions).*

131

MANAGING THE JOB

Too much to do and too little time in which to do it—this is a sure recipe for job-induced stress. An enormous amount of frustration can be avoided by managing time and people wisely.

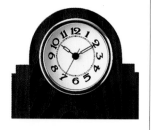

Time management
Sensible scheduling of your time is the key to working efficiently and cutting out unnecessary stress.

Keeping informed
You will work better if you communicate well with colleagues both above and below your job level.

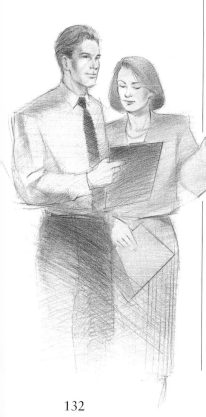

Stress-management experts have identified four qualities in those people who cope best with a difficult work situation: commitment to chosen tasks, viewing problems as challenges rather than difficulties, believing in one's competence to cope in any crisis, and positively welcoming change. You can reduce a large amount of the work pressure you face by altering your attitudes toward your job to match these qualities, but more important you can also adopt certain practical measures to make your working life easier.

Some common stress factors at work are time related, for instance, setting unrealistic targets and therefore missing deadlines. Others are people related—disagreements with your colleagues or differences with your boss, for example. By tackling these two areas alone, you could transform what might be a runaway disaster into a controlled, fulfilling experience.

COMMUNICATION

In one study, it was discovered that 48 percent of industrial employees were unsure of their responsibilities. The researchers attributed this to a lack of proper communication with their superiors. These employees also derived less satisfaction from their jobs than those who felt they understood what was expected of them.

A lack of communication can happen anywhere within a company hierarchy. For a business to achieve its goals, those in possession of needed information must pass it on to others, whether superior or subordinate in the work situation.

Managers are responsible for providing essential data and assigning achievable goals to their subordinates. If you find that you are not being given the information you need by your superiors, try suggesting regular meetings, with a circulation of memos and minutes. Meetings help keep everyone informed of developments and can provide opportunities to define roles and assign tasks. They can also provide open forums to discuss problems. A newsletter and bulletin board can also make developments public.

Asking for help and saying no

Many people hate to ask for help, because they believe it implies they cannot cope. However, requesting assistance does not need to be embarrassing. In fact, your status in the eyes of colleagues can be enhanced by how you enlist help. Often, the person being asked feels flattered, as your request indicates a belief in his or her abilities. And it is productive, since you do not waste a lot of time struggling on your own. A well-timed request for assistance can nip a potential problem in the bud.

The same sort of beneficial response can be gained by learning how to say no constructively. The art of refusing to take on extra work, while avoiding being seen as "difficult," is one that demands a certain amount of skill. The best method is to decline the proposal gracefully but then to offer an alternative solution.

PLANNING AHEAD

When looking at the weeks and months ahead, block in about 10 percent of your schedule as free time, so that you can cope with extra tasks that may arise. If there are things that your daily routine currently does not allow for—like impromptu meetings—make time by marking off hours or days in your diary. You should do the same for leisure activities; they are just as important as work. Also, inform those you work with of their deadlines well in advance so that they can manage their time effectively and avoid the need for asking for extensions to complete their tasks.

Setting priorities is another key to time management. It may be pleasant to discuss matters face-to-face with your clients, but is the time-consuming travel involved really worth it? Can the subject be discussed on the telephone? It may be valuable to attend a seminar, but will it fit into your schedule? Are other matters more pressing?

Organizing daily tasks

Set aside some time first thing in the morning to plan your day. List the things that you want to achieve by the evening. Look at them in terms of how much time they will take and how much time you have, and decide what you can reasonably accomplish during the workday. Those jobs that must be carried out should be assigned a high priority and done at the earliest opportunity. If you see that there are too many tasks to do in one day, determine which are less urgent and tackle them later, or delegate them to a subordinate.

Schedule big or important jobs for times when you are most likely to feel fresh and energetic. You can do less vital jobs at other times. For example, if you are a morning person who often feels less energetic after lunch, then get your most difficult tasks over with early in the day. Save routine jobs such as filing or making phone calls for your afternoon slump time. If possible, intersperse boring or tiring jobs with interesting or easy ones.

As often as you can, complete each task before going on to the next one. Similarly, you should not avoid making decisions; unresolved problems are a source of tension. To aid your concentration, remove all papers from your desk except the ones that refer to the task at hand—you do not want to remind yourself of all the other things that need to be done.

Managing people

Even when you have learned to manage your own time and have control of your workload, you will still have to deal effectively with your boss, colleagues, and subordinates. Building a strong rapport with coworkers will make your job easier and much more rewarding.

Bad working relationships increase stress and concerted efforts should be made to repair them. If you allow extra time for talking through problems with colleagues, you

may improve matters. Good alliances provide tremendous support and confidence and should be nurtured. Looking after work relationships—both good and bad ones—is hard work and can be time consuming.

To get your work done you may need to persuade others to stop wasting your time. For although you may be well disciplined and hardworking, others may not be. These people can steal time from you, either by distracting you with their problems or just by stopping in to talk.

One way is to convince inconvenient visitors that meeting them at another time would be of mutual benefit to you both. Dealing with chatterers, who can be the bane of any office, requires courtesy and resolve. Politely say you do not have time to talk now but you will get back to them. Then get on with some work. If they keep talking, pick up the telephone and make a call (it does not matter to whom); they will not hang around long. So that you do not hurt their feelings, make time to talk when it is more convenient.

TIME MANAGEMENT

If you arrive at work early, leave late, and still take work home, you are likely, if it goes on for too long, to become stressed out. This could lead to a physical illness, a mental breakdown, or total burnout. Learning to manage time correctly can help you avoid these problems.

▶ *Organize your timetable well ahead. For example, if certain meetings are a regular occurrence, record them weeks or months ahead on your calendar.*

▶ *Allow space between projects in case they take longer than expected, and to give yourself time to recover physically and psychologically.*

▶ *If your work piles up, ask your boss to remove or reschedule something from your workload.*

▶ *You could also suggest that it would be possible for you to do the job with additional time or resources. Or you might nominate someone else who has a particular interest or talent in that area. At all times, you should emphasize that you do not want to risk jeopardizing the work you have in progress.*

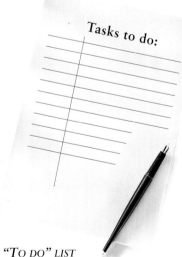

Tasks to do:

"TO DO" LIST
Write down all the tasks you must complete and by when, and keep an ordered account of the point you have reached during the day.

Public Speaking

There are numerous techniques you can learn that will help you give clear, impressive, and successful presentations without any visible signs of nervousness. Time spent in practicing these simple skills will be time well spent.

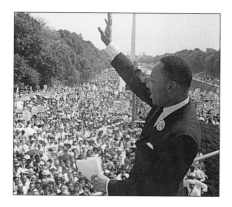

MARTIN LUTHER KING
The greatest public speakers often strike a chord with their audiences by sharing personal experiences.

For most of us, the mere thought of giving a speech is enough to cause numerous symptoms of stress. Instead of running from the anxiety, channel that adrenaline into preparing your speech. Good preparation and a lot of practice are the keys to more confident and competent speech making.

In order to ensure a smooth presentation, you should do the following. Be sure that you cover all the necessary points in your speech. Rewrite any difficult or untidy phrases—you don't want to stumble over your words. Your cards or notes must be legible and in order; if they're not, rewrite and reorganize them. Check that all your visual aids are working; slides or flip charts should be correctly positioned.

BE YOUR OWN AUDIENCE

If you go through your presentation in front of a mirror you may soon see certain areas of your approach that others could find distracting. Do you slouch or lean to one side? Do you scratch your chin too often, or frown, or sniff, or stumble over a particular phrase? Do your clothes hang untidily? Are these aspects that need to be worked on, or are they slight enough to be ignored?

GOLDEN RULES OF PUBLIC SPEAKING

For a successful presentation, follow the three golden rules of public speaking, devised by Dale Carnegie, author of the classic book *The Quick and Easy Way to Effective Speaking.*

▶ *Tell them what you are going to talk about (give a brief overview of your speech).*
▶ *Tell them (present your speech).*
▶ *Tell them what you told them (summarize the key points).*

USING PROMPTS
Practicing often enough will help you memorize most of what you want to say so that you can use your cue cards solely as prompts.

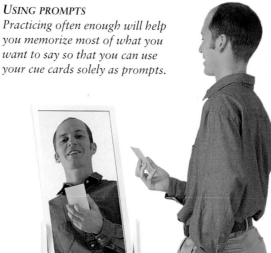

Compose your face to look relaxed and comfortable.

Stand up straight, but do not tense your shoulders or neck.

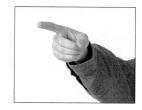

A POINTER
Use your hands to draw attention to your visual aids or to underline certain statements.

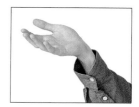

A COMMUNICATOR
An open hand is very reassuring and it also indicates trust, reason, and simplicity.

SPEAKING IN PUBLIC

Try to talk on a subject you know well or one you feel comfortable with. Knowing your material well is essential to building your confidence.

Some people find public speaking much easier if they are talking on behalf of others, such as their company or fellow employees, and not about themselves. Always keep your audience in mind. The majority of speeches are designed to pass on information, so be sure you understand who your listeners are and what they would want to know.

BREATHING EXERCISES

Stressful situations can cause breathing to become fast and shallow, making effective speaking all but impossible. To combat this, do these breathing exercises a few minutes before your speech. They will help you relax and keep your breathing steady and even throughout.

INHALING
Place your right hand index and middle fingers on your forehead. Close your left nostril with your ring finger. Inhale through your right nostril.

When giving a speech, maintain eye contact with your audience. Note cards are useful, but be sure that they are in order. Visual aids like charts, slides, and overhead projectors relieve you of some of the attention, but too many images can be confusing and too much equipment can be distracting.

For good voice projection, practice speaking slightly louder than usual, but do not shout. Talk at a slower pace so your audience can follow you more easily.

EXHALING
Release your left nostril and close your right nostril with your thumb. Exhale through the left nostril. Repeat the sequence.

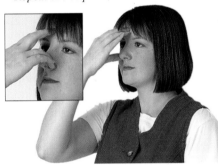

VISUALIZING SUCCESS

Visualization involves making a mental movie of all the various steps involved in a potentially stressful task (see page 41). The goal is to imagine all the steps being performed perfectly. Many athletes use visualization to prepare for competition, but it can be tailored to help in any situation. In one sense, visualization offers you the chance of a dress rehearsal where no one will spot any mistakes except you. At the same time, a positive vision can give you the confidence to take things further. If you visualize your audience enjoying your speech, for instance, it may help you over an

awkward moment in your presentation. Here are some guidelines for using visualization.

▶ *Sit in a comfortable position in a place free of noise and distractions; shut your eyes and relax. Breathe deeply and evenly.*

▶ *Imagine yourself standing in front of your audience. In your mind's eye, try to see as many details as possible. If there will be people that you know and like, concentrate on them.*

▶ *Imagine successfully giving your speech. See the audience enjoying it, and feel your own pleasure at how well you did.*

▶ *Repeat the process until you feel completely confident.*

PREVENTING ANXIETY

Some people become acutely anxious when asked to give a public presentation, and suffer from excessive blushing, rapid heartbeat, shaky legs and hands, and tightness in the chest. Stress-reduction techniques can help to relieve these symptoms.

Behavior therapy can sometimes help allay the fear of public speaking. In this approach, anxious people are taught relaxation techniques, then encouraged to use them while imagining what they most fear: giving a speech. Once clients gain confidence, therapists urge them to give a real speech.

Homeopathy can provide treatment for acute anxiety. A homeopath may prescribe *Gelsemium*, a remedy derived from yellow jasmine. Among the symptoms that it is said to relieve are general nervousness, fears and phobias accompanied by trembling and the need to pass urine, and the inability to sleep because of excitement.

For severe anxiety attacks, your doctor may prescribe a beta-blocker, a drug that blocks some of the effects of adrenaline. It can be taken for a very brief time, but it is not suitable for asthmatics. Tranquilizers can also be prescribed for relief from anxiety.

HERB FOR CALMNESS
A remedy made from Rhus toxicodendron, *a North American species of poison ivy, is used by homeopaths to calm nerves, ease restlessness, and reduce irritability.*

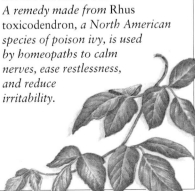

WORK UPHEAVALS

A job provides income, status, and often a social life. Unless handled skillfully, taking a leave of absence or losing a job can upset not only financial security but also a sense of purpose.

Most men and an increasing number of women spend a great proportion of their waking lives at work. (Almost 100,000 hours in all if you start at age 18 and retire at 65.) Studies have shown that people who have supportive relationships at work are less anxious, less depressed, and are ill less often than those who do not work nor have similar supportive relationships. How then does loss of work affect people? Does it matter if the decision not to work was made by the worker?

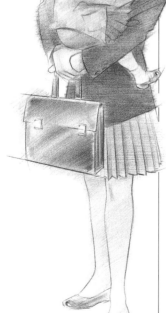

PARENTS AT WORK
Working while raising children demands organization and determination. When managed well, it can be beneficial to everyone.

MATERNITY LEAVE
More and more women are going back to work after having a baby. For many it is not an option; they have to work to support their families. The majority of mothers who work have to make difficult child-care choices (see page 94). Most larger companies have a policy regarding maternity leave—they usually give women between six and eight weeks of paid leave. In the United States, Congress passed the Family and Medical Leave Act, which states that a mother or father who works in a company with more than 50 employees can take up to 13 weeks of unpaid leave. During this time, the employer must continue health care coverage for the employee, and upon the employee's return , provide the same job or a comparable one. In Canada, workers are given up to 41 weeks of maternity leave with 60 percent of pay.

Having a baby is a major milestone that affects every facet of life. For a start, there is the physical ordeal of giving birth and caring for a newborn. There is also the emotional impact a baby can have on a marriage and other family members. Finally, there are the added financial concerns of raising a child and paying for child care. Taking care of a newborn in the first few weeks requires tremendous stamina. For many new mothers, the world of work is all but forgotten in the joy of their new duties. For others, the workplace is sorely missed.

TO RETURN TO WORK OR QUIT
Before the birth of a child, mothers and fathers need to assess their priorities. Can the family get by on one paycheck? Does the mother want to take time off from her career to care for the child? Does the father? Would her company let her work part time? Would his? What type of child care do they want? Is there good day care nearby? Before parents answer any of these questions they should consider how stressful their work is. If the mother's job calls for long hours and lots of deadlines, then caring for a new baby will add a great deal to the family's already high stress levels. This is especially true if the baby needs special attention because of a health problem. It might be wiser to ask for a new assignment for the first few months after returning to work. Should the mother's job be fairly low-key, then managing a new baby, even a difficult one, will be easier. The important thing is to get as much support as possible from the family and employer. Taking care of an infant is very hard work. A new mother should ask for help before the stress gets too high.

Choosing when to return to work can be difficult. Most experts advise mothers of newborns to wait until they feel securely bonded, that is, attached to their baby. Bonding is a mysterious process. For some mothers it occurs at the moment of birth, for others it takes a little longer.

STAYING AT HOME
Many women feel guilty about working instead of remaining at home and taking care of their children. Careful planning can help to ease a woman's return to work and

ensure that both the baby's and mother's needs are met. It's important not to overestimate one's capacity to perform logistical miracles, and to keep in mind personal needs as well as those of the child. Consider joining a group of other mothers to share problems and discover solutions. Negotiate with your partner so that housekeeping duties can be divided equally.

It is reassuring for parents to know that, according to research, the children of working mothers grow up to be confident and well adjusted as long as their parents give them love and attention at predictable times and leave them in charge of caregivers who make them feel secure.

Some women choose to stay at home full time so they have more time and energy for their families. Some choose to wait until they feel that their children are old enough

LEADING U.S. WORK-RELATED DISEASES AND ILLNESSES

According to a study by P.L. Bolakoff in *Issues and Trends in Health,* the greater number of work-related diseases and injuries arise from blue collar jobs, but there has been an increasing shift to white collar stress-related disorders. Work-related disorders include:

▶ *Occupational lung diseases: asbestosis, byssinosis, silicosis, pneumoconiosis (coal workers), lung cancer, occupational asthma.*

▶ *Musculoskeletal injuries: disorders of back, trunk, upper and lower extremities, neck, injury-induced Raynaud's phenomenon.*

▶ *Occupational cancers (other than lung): leukemia, cancers of nose, liver, and bladder.*

▶ *Amputations, fractures, eye loss, lacerations, and fatal injuries.*

▶ *Cardiovascular diseases: hypertension, coronary artery disease, heart attacks.*

▶ *Disorders of reproduction: infertility, spontaneous abortion, birth defects.*

▶ *Neurotoxic (nerve poisoning): peripheral neuropathy, psychoses, extreme personality changes related to toxic exposure.*

▶ *Noise-induced hearing loss.*

▶ *Dermatologic (skin) conditions: scaldings, dermatoses, chemical burns, contusions.*

▶ *Psychological: neuroses, personality disorders, alcoholism, drug dependency.*

to manage without them. For these women, being out of touch with the working world can be stressful. Self-esteem issues can arise, especially if the woman defined herself by her job. Joining a mother's group is a good way to off-load that stress. If possible, arrange to have a sitter for a few hours each day or week. This will give you some time to yourself and allow the baby to learn how to interact with others.

RETIREMENT

After even a few years of hard work, the idea of endless free time for yourself can be very appealing. For many, however, retirement is the long-awaited reward for the years spent working. As with any major life change there are a number of stressful issues to resolve. Decision making is in itself always stressful, and when it comes to one's retirement, there are a great many to make, such as when you want to retire (this is the first and perhaps the most difficult decision), where you want to live, and finally, how you will live.

The key to successful retirement is financial planning. The quality of your retired life will depend to a large extent on how much income you have, and that will depend on what provisions you have made regarding your pension and investments. Ideally, financial planning for retirement should begin years before you leave work. If financial arrangements are left until too late, income could be severely limited. This may require deep cuts in spending or perhaps a move to a smaller, more economical home.

Before you leave the routines of employment behind, it is important to think about what you want to do, if anything, during your retirement. One of the great benefits of retirement is the flexibility it offers, allowing people to take advantage of off-season travel, good weather, special treats that crop up unexpectedly, or simply having time to sit and think. For some retirees, however, the idea of unstructured time can be very unsettling and stressful. If you are worried about how you will spend your days, make a schedule of each day's activities and note the time to be spent on various jobs around the house, sporting events, or volunteer work. Keeping a calendar mimics old work habits and can make the transition to retirement easier.

continued on page 140

KEEPING WELL AT HOME

Many people let good health habits slide when they are not working, leaving themselves open to illness. You can use these strategies to help maintain yourself physically and mentally.

▶ *Avoid living on a diet of convenience foods.*

▶ *Use the extra time you have to shop carefully, choosing the freshest fruit and vegetables and the leanest meat you can find.*

▶ *Take vitamin and mineral supplements, if necessary.*

▶ *Take a brisk walk for at least 20 minutes each day—it's good for the heart and for the circulation.*

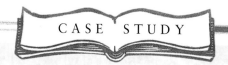
An Out-of-Work Executive

*Losing your job can be devastating. The emotion it generates is often compared
with bereavement. People who have been laid off report feeling a loss of self-worth.
Some see it as shameful and blame themselves. Others are hardier and use their time while
unemployed to finish personal projects and explore new and different types of work.*

Tom is a 50-year-old executive who has worked for an international computer company for the past 20 years. He is a vice president in charge of marketing and supervises a staff of 15. His job is very demanding: it requires long hours and a great deal of international travel.

Eighteen months ago his company merged with another computer company and Tom lost over half his team. His remaining staff were put under pressure to maintain the group's output. Morale plummeted. Tom felt he had let his staff down and buried his guilt in the job. He felt compelled to work harder and increased his time on the road. To allay some of the pressure he felt, he ate more than usual—usually unhealthy foods. He began to smoke again and his alcohol consumption also increased.

Within a few months, Tom's health started to suffer. He began to have difficulty sleeping and complained of headaches, chest pains, and a constant stomach upset. A medical examination revealed that he had both high blood pressure and high cholesterol levels.

His home life was also affected by the strain. Except for the few weekends when he was not overseas on business, he rarely saw his wife Jean or his two sons, aged 12 and 15. Jean, who also worked, had to take on his parenting duties, which caused even more strain in the marriage.

Three months ago, the school psychologist called to say that their younger son was becoming argumentative in class and bullying the younger children in the schoolyard, and urged he be given counseling.

Last week Tom returned from a long trip overseas and learned that his job and his remaining staff were to be eliminated—"effective immediately." He was completely devastated by the news.

FAMILY
Parents' anxieties can be transferred to their children, who then feel insecure about their own lives. These worries can lead to behavioral and psychosomatic problems.

EMOTIONAL HEALTH
Being laid off can bring on self-doubt, just when you need confidence to begin reassessing your skills and abilities.

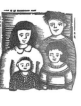

CAREER
It is common for both partners in a marriage to have careers. Often, too little consideration is given to the conflicts of interest this can often cause.

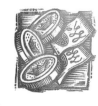

FINANCES
Job loss inevitably brings anxiety over finances, especially if you have a family. Advice from financial experts is essential at this stage.

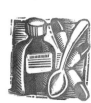

HEALTH
A demanding job, combined with insecurity about employment, can be dangerous to health.

WHAT SHOULD TOM DO?

Tom is in a state of shock and must not make any quick decisions. His company has hired an outplacement firm to help Tom and his staff cope with the dual tasks of dealing with the loss of their jobs and help them look for new ones. It is important that Tom make an appointment with the outplacement counselor immediately. He would also gain some peace of mind if he talked to a financial adviser and found out how much his being laid off will affect his family's material security.

Jean's views and suggestions should also be considered. Tom needs to recognize that she also has suffered from the demands of his career, and that it has taken a heavy toll on their family life.

Tom must try to understand how much his self-esteem is linked to his job, rather than to an inner sense of worth. Instead of viewing being laid off as a tragedy, he could see it as an opportunity to escape from a highly demanding way of life and begin to consider his family's needs and his own well-being.

He also needs to consider some activities, not connected with work, that will build his self-esteem, such as sports or volunteer work. Once he pays some attention to his health, peace of mind, and the happiness of Jean and his sons, he and his family will be able to get back on track.

Action Plan

FAMILY
Recognize that neglect of your family can often lead to tension in a marriage and to problem children. To foster family togetherness, set aside certain weeknights for family-only activities.

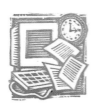

EMOTIONAL HEALTH
Accept that employment with lower status can be just as fulfilling as a high-pressure job, especially if your personal life is given greater emphasis.

CAREER
Visit head hunters and employment agencies to discuss chances of finding new employment. Be clear about what you want from your new job, for instance, working shorter hours. Explore the possibility of becoming self-employed.

HEALTH
Start regular exercise, reduce alcohol consumption, and eat a healthier diet to reduce blood pressure and cholesterol levels. Ask family physician, or family and friends, for ideas for beating insomnia and giving up smoking.

FINANCES
Visit a financial adviser. Discuss the implication of living on a reduced income for both the short and long term. Find out if any grants are available for retraining, or for setting up your own small business.

HOW THINGS TURNED OUT FOR TOM

Tom had four sessions with the outplacement counselor, and many discussions with Jean. At first he was too anxious to focus on anything, and Jean suggested he join a group of unemployed workers who met at their church once a week.

Over time he realized that he had never considered whether he actually liked his job. He discovered he enjoyed marketing computers, but he hated all the traveling. His financial adviser

pointed out that with his severance package and his wife's paycheck, he was financially secure for at least a year. After considering a number of options, he decided to go into partnership with one of his laid-off staff members. They set up a computer consultancy, and soon had their first client. They worked initially out of Tom's home. This arrangement meant Tom could be flexible with his working hours and see more of his sons and his wife.

Although Tom now earns a lot less than previously (partly because he sometimes turns work down), his health has improved considerably. His headaches and chest pains have stopped, and he realizes that they were directly related to all the stresses of his old job.

Tom now enjoys his life and gets immense satisfaction from volunteering at a local charity. He is determined never to allow work to dominate his life again.

Yin and yang balls
Made in China for many
hundreds of years, these
metal balls are thought to
promote good health and
a feeling of well-being.
They are hollow and give
off a high- or low-pitched
ringing sound when
rotated in the hand. They
are available in a variety
of sizes, and as you
become practiced at
manipulating them, you
may progress to larger
ones, or put three or four
in the palm of your hand
at the same time.

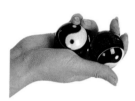

STIMULATING YOUR
ACUPRESSURE POINTS
Using one hand at a time,
move and stretch all your
fingers in sequence to
make the balls revolve
in your palms. This will
stimulate acupressure
points connected to vital
organs, which, it is said,
will help relieve fatigue
and reduce anxiety.

Conflicts at home

Retiring usually means spending more time at home. This can be especially stressful if your partner considers the home his or her domain. Retirees in this situation worry that they will suddenly be under the feet of their partners who, until now, have regarded the home as their own kingdom.

It is important to come to some workable arrangement so that your retirement is not marred by your partner's conflicts with your new lifestyle. If your home is large enough, perhaps you could mark out your own territories. Or you might try sitting down once a week and planning the following seven days so that your partner knows when you will be out of the house and can get on with some of the routine tasks he or she is used to doing alone.

SUDDEN UNEMPLOYMENT

While people can plan for retirement and the positive as well as negative stresses it engenders, finding out that they have been laid off or are being forced to take early retirement usually comes as a shock.

These days layoffs or forced retirements are usually the result of a bad economy or poor management and not anything an employee might or might not have done. Still, human nature dictates that even if you are one of those who are laid off, it is common to think that you are responsible for your unemployment and blame yourself. By incorrectly taking on the responsibility of your layoff you gain a sense of control over the event, but the price is very high, for you are often left with feelings of despair and self-loathing.

Self-blame is debilitating and cuts away at your self-esteem. For this reason alone, counseling is a good idea. Your company may have hired the services of an outplacement firm to help those recently laid off to find other work. Be sure to take advantage of this service. Also consider joining a "job club" to share information with other unemployed workers.

If you have been in the same job for some time, you will probably need to hone your interviewing skills (see page 123). You will also need to learn how to write an effective résumé (see page 122). It's a good idea to create two résumés—one should be chronological for job agencies to review, the other organized around your skills. The latter is particularly useful if you are returning to work after a long absence.

While you are looking for work, you should get in touch with any financial institutions to whom you owe money—most will be sympathetic to your plight. By doing this early on, you may be able to reschedule loan and mortgage payments while you look for employment.

Try to take each day as it comes. Don't let any job rejections discourage you from your goals. Use your free hours to learn new skills. If you have always wanted to change careers, take this opportunity to retrain. Or you could use your spare time to help others by doing volunteer work.

One easy way to earn money and discover whether you are interested in pursuing a new line of work is to register with a temp agency. You can request to work only in industries of your choice.

Some of these agencies offer training in certain skills, such as word processing or bookkeeping, which will help boost your marketability. Temporary employment is an excellent way to supplement fixed incomes with extra money and get a glimpse at how different businesses work. Retirees are finding that temporary work meets a number of their needs. They can choose to work when and where they want, keep a hand in the business world, meet new people, stay active, and earn extra income too.

Pathway to health

There are a number of things to try at home to maintain a positive mental attitude when coping with a change in your work status.

To improve your concentration and ease tension, consider taking a class in yoga (see page 56) or tai chi (see page 36).

Try visualizing (see pages 41 and 147). Not only will it refresh you from the stresses of suddenly being at home, but you can also use it to help you achieve new goals.

Be kind to yourself and set aside time each day to devote to your needs. Practice meditating (see page 42) or simply indulge in a soothing bath with aromatic essential oils (see page 68).

CHAPTER 8

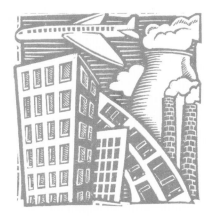

STRESS AND THE ENVIRONMENT

*The frantic pace of modern living
can keep stress levels at a fevered pitch.
Add to this the reports of crime, wars, and other
troubles brought every day into our homes through
the media, and the fight to reduce stress may seem
hopeless. But there are a wealth of strategies
that can help you deal with everyday life.
In this chapter, you'll find helpful tips
to reduce your level of stress.*

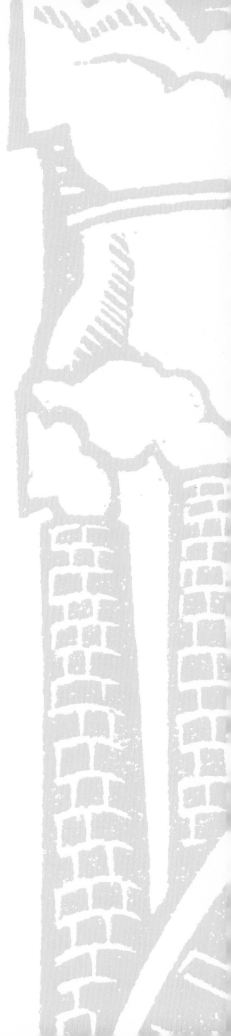

THE WIDER WORLD

Noise, bad weather, pollution, natural disasters—all of these environmental factors create stress, but you can mitigate some of their effects by taking simple, commonsense precautions.

How noise can damage hearing

Sound vibrations funnel into the outer ear and then are registered by the cochlea in the inner ear. The cochlea, a tiny organ shaped like a snail's shell, is lined with some 20,000 groups of delicate hairs that move in response to sound vibrations. This movement is picked up by the auditory nerve, which then conveys the information to the brain. Impaired hearing, even total deafness, can result when sounds are too intense and damage the hairs lining the cochlea.

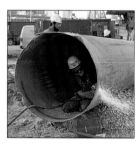

AVOIDING LOUD NOISE Whenever possible, steer clear of places where there is a sustained high volume of noise, such as on a building site where drills are in use.

People have always been at the mercy of political and social change as well as threats from the natural world around them. But today, the plethora of noisy vehicles and machines, industrial water and air pollution, coupled with the sheer pace of modern life, contributes to keeping stress levels very high. Add to these the barrage of worldwide wars and disasters, and it seems that people in contemporary society are subject to more stress-inducing situations than those in many previous ages.

ENVIRONMENTAL FACTORS

Sometimes the impact of the environment on the health of the body's systems is obvious. For example, we now recognize that there are direct links between asbestos and lung disease, and between air pollution and asthma attacks. But the effects of high noise levels seem to be more insidious and take place over a longer period of time.

In the Western world, where many older people show significant hearing loss, it has long been assumed that the decline in the ability to hear was a normal result of aging. But evidence for the contrary has been provided by studies of several preindustrial tribes, such as the bushmen of southern Africa, whose old people show no appreciable loss of hearing. Excessive noise in the modern industrial world is taking its toll. In 1991, scientists at the Harvard Medical School wrote that "a significant amount of hearing loss may be a consequence of a lifetime of exposure to noise rather than an inevitable by-product of growing older." If what they say is true, it makes sense to take

DECIBEL VALUES

Around 80 decibels is the maximum safe limit for hearing (about 130 causes pain in most people). Rock concert music can reach 120 decibels, but sustained noise from common appliances such as vacuum cleaners may pose as much of a risk.

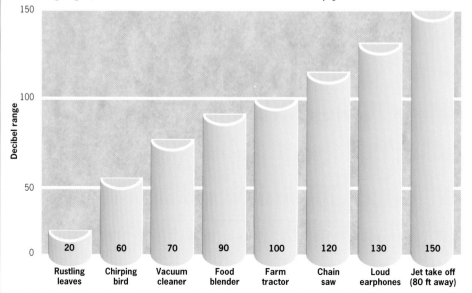

precautions against unnecessary exposure. If you are using a portable tape deck with earphones, for example, keep the volume low. If you are outdoors at an airport when a jet is landing or taking off, cover your ears. When operating a vacuum cleaner or hair dryer, wear earplugs.

The indirect effects of noise

Continual loud noise can cause other problems besides hearing loss. The incessant sounds of sirens and heavy traffic or power mowers and leaf blowers keep a person's body in a constant state of arousal. Just as visible danger provokes a heightened awareness response, noise acts on the autonomic nervous system, raising levels of adrenaline and noradrenaline and increasing heart and breathing rates. These effects continue even when you become so used to certain noises you sleep through them. Research shows that people who live close to airports suffer more than average from such stress-linked ailments as anxiety and high blood pressure, and their use of sedatives is higher.

Fortunately, many government agencies are now monitoring sound levels in problem areas, setting restrictions, and taking action against offenders. You can do your part by supporting and adhering to local ordinances against excessive noise. You can also limit the amount of noise entering your home by installing double- or triple-pane windows and heavy draperies. Consider, too, buying a white noise machine, which modifies the effects of intrusive noises by adding a soothing overlay of sound, such as ocean waves.

Weather and natural disasters

Gloomy skies can mean depressed moods, and for some people, the reduced number of daylight hours during winter can lead

DID YOU KNOW?

Before a thunderstorm, air is low in negative ions; afterward, it is high in them. This may account for the heavy feeling that precedes a storm and the freshness that usually follows. Warm, dry winds, such as the Chinooks in the Rockies, the Santa Ana in southern California, and the Föhn in the northern Alps, are all low in negative ions and are renowned for their ability to make people feel depressed.

Caught in a storm

If you find yourself caught in a thunderstorm while outdoors, look for a sheltered hollow away from trees. If you are in open country, lie flat on the ground. Never shelter under trees or beside a car; both are excellent conductors of lightning. However, if you are in a car, you are safe, because the tires will ground electricity. If you are at home, unplug the television and avoid using the telephone.

SEASONAL AFFECTIVE DISORDER (SAD)

The depression that many people suffer during the winter months is due to the activity of the pineal gland, which is located deep within the brain. It responds to daylight through nerve fibers connecting it to the eyes. As the sun goes down, it begins to release the hormone melatonin, stopping again when the sun comes up. Melatonin is believed to affect the body's circadian (daily) rhythms. Because there is less sunlight during the winter, melatonin levels are at their highest, and high levels suppress some of the body's functions. In some people, this results in depression, anxiety, and lethargy—symptoms which make up the syndrome known as seasonal affective disorder, or SAD. Women suffer from it four times more often than men, although the reason is unknown.

Most sufferers find that their symptoms can be relieved by spending a few hours each day sitting in front of a special light box. This box emits a bright, white, full-spectrum fluorescent light with enough intensity to imitate summer daylight. This tricks the pineal gland

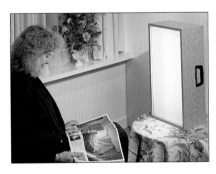

LIGHT THERAPY
Light boxes can trick the pineal gland into producing less melatonin, and provide relief for SAD sufferers.

into producing less melatonin. Most people show improvement within a few days of starting treatment. Doctors also suggest that sufferers spend as many daylight hours as possible outdoors during the winter. In extreme cases, sufferers have moved to sunnier climates.

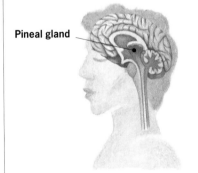

Pineal gland

THE PINEAL GLAND
The body's circadian rhythms, also known as biorhythms, are governed by secretions of the pineal gland.

The "Big One"

Earthquake tremors are experienced not only directly—as when overhead lights sway or cracks appear in walls— but also indirectly. The tremors produce sub-sonic vibrations that can have unsettling effects on the brain, resulting in feelings of anxiety and foreboding even when there is no physical evidence of earth movement.

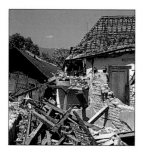

UPHEAVAL
If you live in a known earthquake-prone area, do everything you can to prepare for one, so that you, your home, and your car will sustain the least damage.

to seasonal affective disorder (SAD), more commonly known as the winter blues (see page 143), a medically recognized condition that affects up to one in five people.

Hurricanes, floods, earthquakes, and volcanic eruptions exact dramatic tolls of death and destruction. The predictions of an impending disaster can cause a feeling of helplessness in many people and place them under an additional psychological stress. Knowing emergency procedures and taking sensible precautions can go far toward helping them regain a sense of control.

If you live in an area that is subject to tornadoes, hurricanes, earthquakes, or flooding, you should always keep on hand a battery-powered radio and flashlight with fresh batteries, candles, some nonperishable foods, bottles for water, and a first-aid kit. In addition, plywood and plastic sheeting are useful in hurricane territory.

To limit household damage from an earthquake, anchor the tops of bookcases with L-shaped brackets attached to wall studs, and use a flexible gas-line connector on a stove or a laundry appliance. You can also stabilize a water heater by wrapping it with steel plumber's tape and attaching the tape to wall studs.

Pollution

Air pollution is a concern in many nations today. Heavy automobile and truck traffic, for example, seriously affects air quality in urban areas, and problems are compounded in industrial cities. In some places, up to 40 percent of school-age children who live near major roads suffer from asthma or other chronic respiratory problems. Stringent emission standards and lead-free gasoline plus the limiting of wood burning have all helped to improve the air in some regions. You can do your part by strictly adhering to the air-standard ordinances in your area.

The quality of water varies enormously from one region to another. Industrial and domestic waste products and detergents and nitrates that are used in agriculture get into water supplies through seepage from leaky pipes and uncontrolled runoff into streams and ditches. The dumping of chemicals into lakes, rivers, and oceans plus accidental oil spills from cargo ships have resulted in major ecological disasters. Some situations are improving because of effective fines for large-scale polluters or mandates that they finance a cleanup. Individuals can also help by not using toxic chemicals in their gardens or dumping refuse from their boats.

PURIFYING YOUR WATER

If you are concerned about the quality of your tap water, you can call your municipal water company for a free test, or ask them for the latest monitoring results. If your water comes from a well, you will have to pay for testing.

One of the first things to look for is coliform bacteria, which would indicate pollution from sewage. If it is found you must boil all drinking and cooking water until the situation has been corrected. High levels of copper, iron, chloroform (a by-product of chlorination), or nitrates can be harmful. The presence of *any* lead, mercury, or arsenic is dangerous. Consult a water-treatment expert for a solution.

A pH test is also a good idea. If your water is found to be acidic (pH below 7), it can corrode pipes and leach metals, such as those listed above, into the water.

A carbon water filter (see right) will remove chemicals, odors, and a bad taste,

but not lead. Filter cartridges are available for lead removal; a distiller will remove lead and microorganisms as well, but not ordinary chemicals. These devices must be regularly maintained.

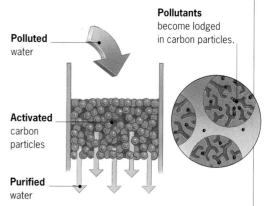

Pollutants become lodged in carbon particles.

Polluted water

Activated carbon particles

Purified water

FILTERED WATER
Carbon water filters work by passing water slowly through charcoal permeated with tiny channels, to which the pollutants will stick.

THE WORLD STAGE

The media reports of wars, hostage taking, and famines around the world are more graphic and immediate than ever and help perpetuate negative images and attitudes. This continual assault on people's sensitivities can lead to what is known as compassion fatigue as well as depression about the state of the world and an increased sense of helplessness in the face of all of these horrors. Nevertheless, by maintaining an awareness of what is happening in the world around you and by learning to appreciate improvements where they do occur, you will develop a greater ability to retain realistic expectations and to avoid stress-making disappointments.

Bad news

Crime statistics are often among the most worrying kinds of news. The sensationalist reporting of relatively rare cases, such as those concerning serial killers or kidnappers, sells newspapers and increases television audiences. It also results in these crimes appearing to be much more of a risk than they actually are.

In 1990, for example, a total of 67 children were killed in the UK—a disturbing figure, but not high enough to constitute a wave of infanticide in a population of more than 50 million. In the US the percentage was higher, but the reported 888 child murders took place in a nation of more than 250 million people. As a consequence of largely unwarranted fears, many children today are more restricted and monitored than in the past, despite the fact that child-related crime has shown little increase.

The evidence for any real increase in the rate of crime is not necessarily supported by the rise in reported cases. In recent years the apparent escalation in rape, for example, is to some extent the result of the larger numbers of courageous women who are now reporting it to the police. The statistics may simply be reflecting a truer picture of what was actually happening before.

Although the tables of facts and figures are scarcely much comfort for those who have encountered or fear to suffer the effects of crime, it does put the true issue into a less perilous perspective. Violent crime, which primarily affects young males, is mainly recorded among groups on the shadowy fringes of law-abiding society.

Statistics for nonviolent crimes against property tell a similar story of fear outrunning the peril. Older people are particularly prone to worries about burglary, leading them to feel that they are prisoners in their own homes. Yet elderly people are not high on the list of victims among the thousands every year who suffer break-ins. In fact, the figures demonstrate that the most vulnerable groups in the community—women, children, and the elderly—are statistically the least likely to be affected by crime.

They also show that the lion's share of statistics is taken up by the less mysterious or sinister aspects of criminal activity. The majority of people are more likely to deal only with crime that involves no violence or confrontation (car theft and pickpocketing, for example). Violence, or the threat of it, is almost universally domestic—generally the result of open and long-running conflicts between spouses or members of the same family, in which emotional antagonisms spill over momentarily into a more physical form of expression.

It is sensible not to expose yourself to unnecessary dangers, and any precaution you take is good. But becoming aware of the myths as well as the facts about crime will help you assess the real risks you face so you can make better decisions about how to deal with them. Listed on page 146 are a number of steps you can take to make yourself less vulnerable and reduce your risk of becoming another crime statistic. It is better to be safe than sorry.

> ## *Pathway to health*
> Psychotherapists and others who work with people under stress suggest that the degree to which individuals feel in control of their lives significantly affects how they react to stress. People need to believe that they can influence their environment. If you feel bothered by things that appear to be out of your control, you may find that it would be beneficial to consult a psychotherapist. He or she will help you to come to a clearer understanding of why you are feeling this way, and enable you to put your troubles in perspective.

Is your child safe?
With so much crime being reported in the media, parents no longer feel secure in allowing their children the freedom they themselves once enjoyed. A child cannot always be under the protecting supervision of a parent, however, so make sure yours understands the danger of strangers offering a ride or candy. All children should also know their own address and telephone number as well as the name and telephone number of a family friend or relative.

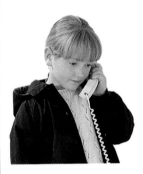

SAFETY MEASURES
As early as possible in your child's life, show him or her how to use the telephone, and particularly how to make emergency calls.

SAFETY OUTSIDE

Safety on the streets is everyone's responsibility; we should all be alert and prepared to take action to prevent crimes and the stresses they induce.

Face-to-face with potential violence

Because one of the most effective deterrents against assault is to make the assailant feel you might be able to ward off an attack, looking self-assured can help reduce your vulnerability.

Enrolling in a self-defense class will give you the confidence and ability to walk, talk, and behave in an assertive, purposeful manner.

Some people who have escaped attack have spoken of the value of "dissipating the atmosphere" of potential violence. This is done by keeping calm and avoiding sudden movements when menaced by an assailant. If possible, try to maintain eye contact, and talk in a matter-of-fact voice. Should the encounter escalate into violence, it is best to comply with the demands of the attacker.

While violent assault is a rarity, the fact is that most people will eventually have some experience with a minor crime such as theft or vandalism. Being a victim can cause you to have less self-confidence and harbor bad memories for weeks, perhaps even months afterward. It is therefore wise to consider realistically and carefully what you as an individual can do to keep feelings of helplessness from spilling over into your daily life. A good start is to contact your local police precinct and ask them to advise you on any risky areas in your neighborhood that you should avoid. The police should also have information on local groups such as Neighborhood Watch and women-only taxi services. In addition, many police departments have a crime prevention officer who is available to discuss safety measures.

You should also think about what actions you can take to protect yourself and your family outside the home, whether you are on foot (see below) or in your car. When driving in a risky neighborhood, especially at night, lock the doors, keep windows shut, and stow valuable items, such as purses and cellular phones, out of sight. If you suspect you are being followed, drive to a well-lit area, where there are people around, and ask for help. Also, if you see what appears to be an accident or someone tries to flag you down, consider the situation very carefully before stopping. It might be safer to drive on until you find a convenient phone from which to report what you have seen.

Campaigning for improved street lighting can also contribute to building collective responsibility for security with neighbors and increasing your personal sense of safety.

BECOMING STREETWISE

One of the most effective ways to prevent yourself from becoming another crime statistic is to think strategically and avoid presenting an open invitation. Being aware of your surroundings can help you to steer clear of trouble.

▶ *If you carry a purse, use one with a shoulder strap and wear it slung across your body.*

▶ *When shopping, take only as much cash as you expect to need and handle it discreetly.*

▶ *Travel on busy, well-lit streets. Plan your route to avoid empty underpasses and dark streets and alleys.*

▶ *Be sure of your route before setting out, so you won't have to ask for directions.*

▶ *When traveling by train or subway, avoid sitting in an empty compartment. If the one you are in empties, move to another.*

▶ *If you think someone is paying you too much attention, do not acknowledge the person but move to a place where there are other people.*

▶ *If somebody is following you, cross the road and, if necessary, go into a shop or knock at a house.*

▶ *Walk facing the flow of traffic so that a car cannot pull up behind you unnoticed.*

▶ *If you carry an alarm or whistle, be sure to hold it in your hand. It will be of no use buried at the bottom of your purse.*

▶ *Always have your key ready as you approach your home or your car.*

▶ *Take a self-defense course to increase your confidence.*

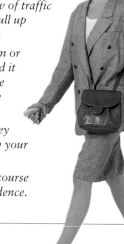

Visualization

The ability to free your mind of distracting thoughts in order to achieve a goal or cope with a stressful situation is a vital skill in combating the pressures of life. It works by letting your imagination take you to calm and restful places.

You can greatly enhance the effects of progressive relaxation (see page 39) by visualizing an idyllic haven and then placing yourself in this imaginary picture. The exercise will bring mental calmness and further reduce physical tension.

After progressively relaxing all your muscles, start saying the words 'serene,' 'safe,' 'calm,' 'relaxed' over and over again in your head. Focus on them, and when other thoughts try to enter your mind, gently push them away. Then imagine an appealing place; it could be a favorite room, a forest glade, lush island, lake, beach, or mountainside. It may be a location that you know or just a product of your imagination. The key is that it should be a spot where you can feel happy and secure.

Perform your visualization in a comfortable position in a place where you will not be disturbed.

A TIME AND A PLACE

To shut out distractions, choose a quiet, dimly lit place in which topractice visualization, or positive thinking techniques. Ask your family not to disturb you for half an hour.

Wear loose-fitting, comfortable clothing, and lie down on a very firm bed, or on a blanket laid on the floor, with a thin cushion under your head. Alternatively, you can sit in a high-backed armchair that will provide some support for both your head and back.

PRACTICAL VISUALIZATION EXERCISE

Take a relaxing mental vacation with these simple steps. Close your eyes and imagine that you are eating a ripe peach. You will find that your mouth waters, such is the power of imagination to affect your body. Now choose a pleasant haven where you would like to relax, and visit it in your mind. Smell the smells, feel the air, hear the sounds, notice all the sights. Make a practice of visiting your retreat regularly and you will reap the benefits.

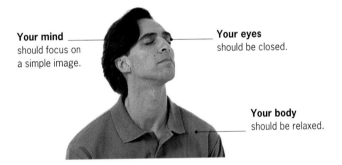

Your mind
should focus on a simple image.

Your eyes
should be closed.

Your body
should be relaxed.

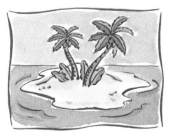 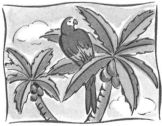 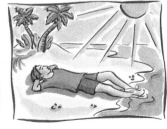 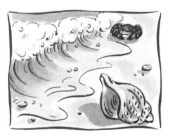

1 *Once you have chosen your haven, begin examining it in your mind's eye. If you have selected a tropical island, you might see expanses of sandy beach fringed by blue sea, and perhaps a palm tree outlined against a cloudless sky.*

2 *Then look at the scene in more detail. There may be a few puffs of cloud, flecks of white foam on the waves, or perhaps a boat on the horizon, some shells along the shore, and possibly a colorful parrot perching in the palm tree.*

3 *Listen to the sounds of your sanctuary. These might include the splashing of the waves against the shore, the squawking of the parrot, the chirping of other birds, or the whisper and rustle of the palm's fronds in the breeze.*

4 *Now feel the fine sand run through your fingers, the warm sun on your skin, and the silkiness of the ripples of water tickling your feet. Imagine you can pick up a beautiful shell, and when you hold it to your ear, you can hear the sound of the sea.*

MANAGING TRAUMA

In the event of a crime, accident, or full-scale disaster, knowing what the most common human reactions are can give you and those you love emotional protection.

HOW TO SURVIVE A TRAUMA

Traumas are deeply personal experiences and reactions to them differ, depending on the nature of the event and the personality of the individual involved. But there are some practical steps that can help.

▶ *Allow plenty of time for sleep and rest.*

▶ *Don't bottle up your feelings: talking or crying can bring relief.*

▶ *Let the event work itself through a little at a time. Allow yourself to think about it, and do not be afraid of any bad dreams that you may experience.*

▶ *Keep to your usual daily routine as much as possible, but take special care when driving or carrying out difficult or stressful tasks.*

▶ *Don't isolate yourself; be with family and friends when you can.*

At times of major crises, reactions of shock, fear, and anger are very common, and they are often followed by feelings of sadness, helplessness, and guilt. But less obvious consequences—physical as well as psychological—may also follow, even after some delay. Such symptoms may be indicators of post-traumatic stress disorder, or PTSD.

PTSD can be triggered by any distressing traumatic event outside the normal range of experience. A natural disaster, war, or, more commonly, a serious assault, near-drowning, or a fire or traffic accident may cause anyone who experiences the event, and even those witnessing it, to develop PTSD.

Consequences of PTSD

The event may be reexperienced in the form of unprompted memories. There may be disturbed sleep or nightmares, or even vivid flashbacks during waking hours, when sufferers feel and react as if the events were taking place all over again.

Sufferers sometimes undergo an emotional numbing as well. They may lose interest in their hobbies, their work may deteriorate because they find it difficult to concentrate, and their memory might become poor. The traumatic events could become unreal to them, seeming to be like dreams, and they may begin to feel detached from the rest of the world. Personal relationships can suffer, often as a result of the victims' desires to avoid anything that symbolizes or recalls the traumas they have endured. As a consequence, they may begin using or increase their consumption of alcohol or narcotics.

Unpleasant physical sensations, such as headaches and abdominal pains, are common, too. In addition, there may be periods of palpitations, trembling, breathing difficulties, dizziness, tightening in the chest, menstrual disorders, nausea, or diarrhea.

As symptoms can occur some time after the actual events that trigger them, the link between the symptoms and trauma may not be obvious. If they remain unrecognized and untreated, these symptoms have the power to destroy lives by changing the sufferer's personality and damaging social and family relationships. It is important to seek immediate help from health professionals and support groups when symptoms of stress from a traumatic event first begin to surface.

Treating trauma

At the heart of all prevention and treatment of PTSD is the sharing of the traumatic experience with others. One approach is to talk through the pain with people who have undergone a similar trauma. While much relief can be gained by discussing a trauma with fellow survivors, complex psychological issues such as survivor's guilt or blaming oneself can arise. If this occurs, one should turn to a psychologist or psychotherapist trained in treating PTSD as soon as possible.

One approach used frequently is debriefing, in which sufferers are helped to counter any instinctive feeling to shut the event out, because of fears that they may have of losing control. Instead, they are encouraged to let the reality of the event work itself through, by talking about the experience with sympathetic listeners. The debriefing may take the form of individual or group discussions, and is usually carried out as soon as possible after the event.

If the shock and trauma are deep or the victim is particularly vulnerable, then more intensive counseling may be necessary. As well as going over all of the events of the traumatic experience in great detail, the counselor and sufferer investigate how these events have affected his or her physical and emotional responses and ways of thinking, reacting, and coping with things in general.

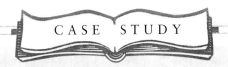

Post-Traumatic Stress Victim

The effects of a traumatic event are not always felt immediately. Both emotional reactions and physical symptoms can occur weeks or months later, and their link with the crisis may not be clear. Yet if symptoms of post-traumatic stress disorder (PTSD) go untreated, they can be more incapacitating and longer lasting than a physical injury.

Nick, a young engineer, had just been promoted to a more responsible position, when he was attacked by a gang of drunken youths after a night out. While the attack was violent, and he sustained severe bruising, he escaped before suffering any major injury. A couple of weeks later, however, he had trouble getting to sleep and began to experience disturbing flashbacks. As the days passed, feelings of anxiety, accompanied by palpitations, sometimes overwhelmed him. To escape these feelings, he is now drinking heavily, which is having a bad effect on his relationship with his girlfriend, Anna. At work, he is irritable with colleagues and is finding it hard to concentrate, so he makes repeated mistakes.

WHAT SHOULD NICK DO?

Nick must accept that he has a problem and seek professional help. Simply making the decision to do this will boost his confidence.

During debriefings by his counselor, Nick should resist the temptation to bury the experience. By going over the events of that evening in detail and facing up to what he felt during the attack, he will realize how natural his reactions are. When he has understood how the experience has affected him, he should talk to his girlfriend and explain the reasons for his antisocial behavior. He should also take steps to reduce stress levels by taking on less work for the time being, looking after himself physically, and having some time off to relax.

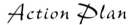

Action Plan

EMOTIONAL HEALTH
Contact a support group to find out what kind of help is available and share the experience with others who have suffered similarly. Temporarily adopt a slower pace of life, with plenty of time for rest.

PARTNERS
Stop burying the crisis, allow feelings to surface, and talk to Anna. Ask for her understanding and support while recovering from the effects of the attack.

WORK
Ask for a leave of absence or to have his amount of work reduced temporarily.

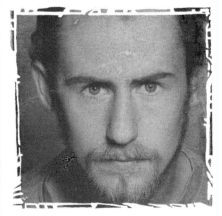

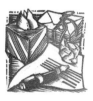

EMOTIONAL HEALTH
A refusal to face up to feelings of anxiety may result in severe depression and destructive patterns of behavior.

PARTNERS
Lack of communication about distressing issues can cause misunderstandings and result in the breakdown of relationships.

WORK
The feelings that arise from a traumatic episode may interfere with the ability to carry out a job.

HOW THINGS TURNED OUT FOR NICK

Nick contacted a victims' support group, which helped him realize his problems were not unique. He discussed details of the event with a therapist, who encouraged him to confront his memories and look at the emotional turmoil the attack had caused. With the backing of the group, Nick opened up to Anna and was relieved to find she was very sympathetic. Nick became less anxious, and is slowly regaining his old confidence.

TAKING THE STRESS OUT OF TRAVELING

The journey to and from work, whether by car or public transportation, can be full of annoyances that increase stress. Traveling for pleasure can have its stressful side, too.

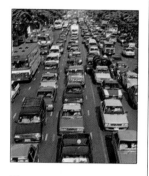

TRAFFIC JAM
Slow-moving traffic is a fact of urban life. Use this time constructively: listen to a recorded book, learn a language on cassette, or just catch up with the news.

Some people enjoy their daily commute to work because it gives them time to become fully alert in the morning or to unwind from the tensions of the day. Others find that their commuting time affects their well-being and they arrive at their destination feeling tense or drained. If you fit the latter category, the suggestions below may help make your commute less harrowing.

DRIVING STRESS

When road conditions are congested, many people, even those who are normally placid, become antagonistic and irritable behind the wheel and succumb to "road rage." This is a blind fury that causes aggressive and reckless driving behavior, such as traveling at high speeds, lane-hopping, jumping the gun at traffic lights, and generally being obstructive or discourteous. Aside from the obvious risk of having an accident, if road rage recurs continually, it can result in long-term health problems such as high blood pressure and heart disease.

If you feel road rage coming on, say to yourself such things as: "I am not the only driver on the road" and "I don't have special rights" or "Whatever that driver did, I've done myself on occasion." Then distance yourself from your predicament by rising above it. Try to think of the situation as an enormous internal combustion engine, where patience, courtesy, and consideration are the oil that keeps the system lubricated and moving. This will help free you from the shackles of anger.

You may have to weigh the consequences of being late for an important business meeting or appointment against those of angering another motorist or having an accident—all clearly stressful prospects. (Of course, the predicament is less likely to arise if you allow enough time for delays.) In the end, it's better to slow down and drive carefully. You will arrive at your destination more relaxed, yet alert.

Public transportation and stress

On public transportation, when delays and overcrowding occur, irritation can be compounded by a sense of inability to control your own fate. Besides having to deal with disgruntled fellow travelers, you must place your fate entirely in the hands of others—drivers, pilots, baggage handlers, or flight controllers. This passive acceptance of such impediments can lead to a buildup of toxins and excessive acidity in the body, and the excess hormones released during stress responses can interfere with the body's

DRIVING AND YOUR HEALTH

Stress while driving can be measured directly by tests of skin resistance (tautness), eye movement (which reveals how much information is being conveyed to the brain), heart rate, and blood pressure. Even very experienced drivers demonstrate a 50 percent increase in these measurements when driving in heavy traffic. And when they have to struggle to read road signs, negotiate traffic circles, or wait at red lights or in traffic jams for long periods, there are corresponding surges in these levels.

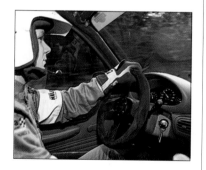

RACING DRIVER STRESS
Tests on racing car drivers have shown sustained heart rates that are 50 percent above normal, peaking in excess of 200 beats per minute. Physical effects may include weight loss, dehydration, and exhaustion.

immune system, leaving it more vulnerable to bacteria and viruses such as the flu.

To make this type of commuting easier on the nerves, carry a good book or magazine to read, so that you can tune out aggravations; or if you do needlecraft, work on a project to make productive use of the time; or use the time to catch up on your paper work. You might also try persuading the company you work for to adopt flextime so that you can travel outside of peak hours.

Safety and emergency measures

The compulsory wearing of seat belts has proved its worth. Statistics from the US National Highway Traffic Safety Administration show that wearing a lap/shoulder seat belt reduces the risk of fatal injury to a front-seat car passenger by 45 percent. A further level of safety is provided by airbags, which can significantly reduce the risk of serious facial and chest injuries for a driver (and front passenger in a dual-bag vehicle).

Making sure that the vehicle you travel in is safe can help reduce stress. It should be serviced regularly and repaired as necessary, with frequent checks especially on brakes and tire conditions and pressure.

If you do have a breakdown, get the car as far off the road as possible, turn on the emergency flashers, and set up flares if you have them. Open the hood and wait in the car until help arrives. If you cannot get the car off the road, you will probably be safer standing on the roadside. If you have a cellular phone (a good traveling companion for dealing with emergencies), you can call for assistance. Otherwise, ask a passing motorist to call for help at the nearest phone or tollbooth.

LONG-DISTANCE TRAVEL

Traveling for extended periods in a car can result in stresses that are very different from those of daily commuting. For most people, long-distance driving is physically exhausting; regular stops are essential to relieve cramped and tense muscles and keep the driver mentally alert. It is surprising how much benefit can be gained from even a short pause in driving.

Long car journeys are made easier with activity. Singing, listening to books on tape, playing word games, following an extended discussion or musical program on the radio, or just talking can help ward off boredom and irritation. Try to avoid any arguments, however, as the stressful atmosphere they generate can distract you and negatively influence your driving, exposing you and your companions to the risk of an accident.

One of the hazards of long-distance travel is that it can lead to drowsiness. Of the 50,000 or so deaths from motor vehicle accidents in the United States each year, 13 percent are caused by drivers falling asleep.

Relax while traveling

Worrying about problems will only increase your stress, so try to steer your thoughts onto more tranquil topics.

If you are a passenger, an inflatable neck pillow will provide comfort and help you to take a nap. When awake, regularly do muscle relaxation exercises, like those below. If you are traveling on public transportation, these can be done discreetly so as not to disturb other passengers.

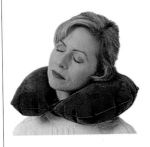

SLEEP PILLOW
An inflatable pillow may help you sleep more easily on a long journey, as it provides support for your neck.

EXERCISES FOR LONG-DISTANCE PASSENGERS

Sitting in an upright position for a long time with limited body movement restricts blood flow and causes stiffness and aches.

These simple exercises can help reduce discomfort and make you feel more alert on arrival at your destination.

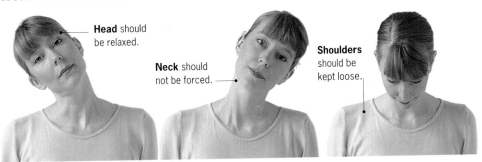

Head should be relaxed.

Neck should not be forced.

Shoulders should be kept loose.

1 *Take a deep breath and slowly lean your head to one side. Rest it gently in this position for three seconds, then exhale.*

2 *Follow the same routine with the other side. Repeat these exercises three times. Do not bounce, rotate, or swivel your neck.*

3 *Bend your head forward; hold for three seconds. Move head to right then left, holding for three seconds on each side. Repeat three times.*

TIPS FOR AIR TRAVEL

Long hours in a confined space can make air travel trying. Here are a few tips to help lessen the stress.

▶ *Wear comfortable, loose clothing; remove shoes and put on slippers or an extra pair of socks.*

▶ *In your hand luggage carry toiletries and a change of underwear in case your baggage is delayed or lost.*

▶ *Avoid alcoholic drinks. The air in the cabin is very dry and causes dehydration. Alcohol will dehydrate you more.*

▶ *Drink plenty of water or fruit juice.*

▶ *Every hour or so, get up and walk the length of the airplane, if possible.*

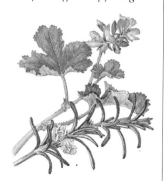

ROSEMARY
AND GERANIUM
The essential oils of these herbs are refreshing and can help alleviate some of the effects of jet lag.

If you find yourself beginning to nod off behind the wheel, the safest solution is to stop as soon as you can and get some sleep. If this isn't possible, open the window and let fresh air blow on your face. Or stop the car and jog around it a few times. Other wake-up ideas are: tuning into a radio station and turning up the volume (with the window rolled up), talking back to a talk-show host, singing loudly, stopping for a cup of coffee and a brisk walk. Also, sitting with an erect posture and having the top of the head pulling the neck and spine as straight as possible will enable blood to flow more freely and encourage wakefulness.

FEAR OF FLYING

According to the US National Transportation Safety Board, flying is one of the safest forms of travel. The systems for controlling traffic are sophisticated, mechanical inspection of planes is regular, and the training of pilots and other crew is demanding. Statistics show that the fatality rate for air travel is negligible compared with other forms of transportation.

Despite the statistics, many people are afraid of flying. Whether or not you are in this group, you will have more peace of mind if you fly with an airline that has a good safety record. Most large, regularly scheduled airlines meet these standards; chartered carriers vary. Also, if possible, fly out of airports that have stringent security checks. Before takeoff, pay attention to the safety briefing presented and read the safety instruction card.

Even if you have a phobia against flying, there is still hope. Psychotherapy, hypnosis, and desensitization courses can do much to reduce these fears by getting you used to all aspects of the flying experience. Joining a support group may also be helpful.

JET LAG

When flying across time zones, it is not uncommon to suffer from an interrupted sleep pattern, irritability, and fatigue, which may last several days. Known as jet lag, this results from disruption of the body's internal clock. The time it takes to recover from it depends on what time the flight left and how many time zones were crossed and in which direction. Crossing one to three time zones takes little adjustment (if the trip is a short one, it might be better to stay on your own time for its duration). Moving across six or seven zones requires much more.

Going from east to west is easier to adjust to if you take a late afternoon or evening flight, stay awake during the flight, then go to bed shortly after you arrive. Traveling west to east, you will lose a vital number of sleep hours on an overnight flight. If you take a daytime flight, then have dinner and go to sleep relatively late in the new time zone, you will be more rested and your time clock will be better adjusted the next day.

If possible, start to readjust your routine several days before your flight—getting up an hour earlier or later and going to bed earlier or later—to mirror what you will need after your journey. Have as little caffeine as possible in the three days prior to departure. Also, eat lightly the day before and during the flight. Allow yourself a day to rest and recover if you have important business to attend to.

Many people suffer from light deprivation when they return from a winter vacation—going from fun in the sun to the artificial light of an office building. Spending time exposed to the sun shortly after landing can help mitigate the effects of jet lag.

VACATION TRAVEL

Getting away on vacation does not necessarily mean that you will be able to leave all your stresses behind. But careful planning can help ensure your trip gets off to a relaxing start and continues that way.

Rather than coping with heavy luggage, take along no more than you absolutely need and pack well in advance. Taking just two basic colors, such as black and white or beige and blue, permits you to mix and match items. Including clothing that can be layered will prepare you to meet varying weather conditions comfortably. Leave out things that you are tempted to take "just in case." When you are flying and planning to check your bag, keep a tote or carry-on bag with toiletries, a change of underwear, all medications, and any items of value.

Plan your route in detail to avoid arguments and anxiety. If you are going by bus, train, or plane, allow plenty of time to get to your departure point and avoid last-minute panics. When flying, choose a schedule that allows enough time to make any connections. If a tight connection is unavoidable, find out what the next available flight will be if you should miss your connection. Also, make a hotel reservation for at least the first night away, and learn as much as you can about your destination to orient yourself without difficulty.

If you are traveling abroad, make sure that you arrive with sufficient foreign currency to pay transportation and tips to your hotel. Include some change, as many bus and taxi drivers will not accept bills in large denominations. If you do not know the language spoken at your chosen destination, buy a traveler's phrase book and practice a few simple phrases to help you with your first few transactions.

Give a neighbor the phone numbers where you can be reached in an emergency, and the numbers of friends or relatives who can deal with unexpected problems. Provide this same person or another trusted friend or relative with a list that contains the numbers of all your credit cards, traveler's checks, and passport if you're going abroad.

In cold weather, make sure that your home is heated well enough to prevent the pipes from freezing. You could also ask a friend or relative to stay there while you are away (or check the newspapers for persons advertising to house sit); this would give you an added sense of security.

In case you are stranded

In many parts of the world, tourists are advised to carry cash, checks, and passports in a fanny pack or a hidden money belt, because travelers tend to stand out from the locals and are frequently vulnerable targets for theft. Despite precautions, thefts still occur. If you become a victim, report the theft immediately to the police; in the case of traveler's checks, notify the company that issued them (be sure to carry the numbers and record of checks cashed separately from the checks themselves). In most cases, you will receive new checks within 24 hours.

If you need some cash, automatic teller machines are widely available today. An alternative is to have a friend or relative wire you some money. Depending on the location, this can usually be transacted at a bank, a traveler's checks agency, or a telegraph office. You might also arrange to have funds transferred from your own bank to a local one.

Star-of-Bethlehem

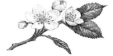

Cherry plum

Clematis

Impatiens

Rock rose

RESCUE REMEDY Extracts from these herbs comprise Rescue Remedy, a popular Bach Flower Remedy.

REMEDIES FOR TRAVEL STRESS

There are a number of practical measures you can take to make travel less stressful for you and your family. For example, to boost your energy and be prepard for possible delayed mealtimes, carry with you such snack foods as nuts, dried fruit, and whole-grain crackers. To prevent dehydration, drink bottled mineral water (you can also use it to brush your teeth if there is any doubt about the local water supply). To accommodate swollen feet when flying, remove your shoes and put on extra socks or slippers. To help you sleep, use earplugs and eyeshades.

Alternative therapists also recommend travel stress remedies (see the list below). You can use these alone or in conjunction with the other measures in this chapter.

HOMEOPATHIC

To minimize the effects of jet lag and aid adjustment when flying through a significant number of time zones, take *Cocculus* 6 for three days before departure. *Arnica* 6 may also ease the transition if taken during the flight and for a couple of days afterward.

AROMATHERAPY

To reduce anxiety before the journey, use rose, juniper, or sandalwood essential oils. To relax you during the journey, use lavender oil. To relieve fatigue after the journey, try rosemary, lemon, geranium, jasmine, or bergamot essential oils. Place two or three drops of oil on a tissue and inhale, or add to your bath, or massage into tired muscles (see page 68).

BACH FLOWER REMEDIES

If you are prone to panic and anxiety—particularly when flying or going on long journeys—place three drops of Rescue Remedy on your tongue every hour before, during, and after the journey (see right).

HERBAL

To help you sleep during the journey, take along a pillow that is filled with lavender, chamomile, lime blossoms, or hops. You can also drink herbal teas, especially chamomile or passion flower tea.

Motion sickness

This condition is caused by changes in speed and direction that upset the delicate balance mechanism in the inner ear, which is responsible for informing the body of its position, movement, and acceleration. The roll and pitch of a ship, the undulations of an airplane in rough weather, and the rotation of amusement park rides can all induce motion sickness in varying degrees.

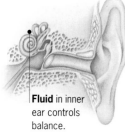

Fluid in inner ear controls balance.

THE INNER EAR
The balance of the fluid-filled, semicircular canals in the inner ear becomes disrupted during motion sickness.

GINGER TEA
Any form of ginger—tea, capsules, preserved, or sticks—helps settle and warm the stomach. For fresh ginger tea infuse one slice of peeled ginger in a cup of boiling water.

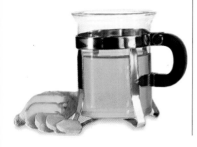

Report a stolen or lost passport to the police as well as the nearest US embassy or consulate. You will need the police report to obtain a new passport. If you have the number of your original passport (better yet, a photocopy of it) or any other proof of citizenship, then you should receive a new passport within a day. But you will have to spend time standing in lines and filling out forms, which will cut into your vacation.

For a lost airline ticket, go to the office of the company that issued it. You will probably have to buy a replacement and then wait for a refund. Policies vary.

Preventing motion sickness

Even seasoned travelers can be affected occasionally by motion sickness. Sometimes anxiety and fatigue make a person more susceptible. Whatever your travel mode, try to remain still enough to give the body's balance mechanism a chance to settle down. If possible, lie on your back. This position has been shown to reduce the incidence of motion sickness by about one-fifth.

Avoid traveling on a full stomach. Eating a snack may settle it, but a large meal will make you feel worse. Do not read or play games that require close focusing; straining your eyes to cope with the uneven bumping of the journey will exaggerate the sense of erratic movement that the brain receives.

HOMEOPATHIC TREATMENT

Depending on your symptoms, take one to three pills an hour to relieve them, until they disappear.

▶ *Cocculus 6* For nausea with giddiness and a metallic taste in the mouth.

▶ *Sepia 6* For nausea aggravated by the smell of food, alleviated by eating.

▶ *Nux vomica 6* For nausea with chills; symptoms relieved by vomiting.

▶ *Petroleum* For nausea accompanied by dizziness, faintness, and cold sweat.

When traveling by airplane, sit toward the front or over the wing for the smoothest ride. Recline your seat and press your head against the headrest. On a ship, stay in the midsection where it is most stable. If you have a cabin, lie down. If you don't, sit on deck or by a window where you can see the horizon to orient yourself.

There are a number of treatments for motion sickness; you may have to try them all to see which one works best for you. Bands are available that put continuous pressure on the wrist acupressure point that alleviates nausea. Patches behind the ears release anti-nausea medication directly into the bloodstream. Ask your pharmacist for advice. A drop of peppermint oil placed on the tongue might also help.

ACUPRESSURE FOR MOTION SICKNESS

If you suffer badly from motion sickness when traveling, help may be at hand. Acupressure can be used to help prevent or alleviate the nausea that is associated with motion sickness (and also morning sickness). Try the methods illustrated below to help make your journey as comfortable as possible.

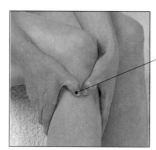

Use both thumbs to massage—the point may feel very tender.

TO PREVENT MOTION SICKNESS
Sitting with feet flat on the floor, find a spot on the outside of your calf 4 to 5 inches below the right knee. Massage it firmly with your thumbs for 20 seconds, breathing deeply. Repeat on the left leg. Do each leg three times.

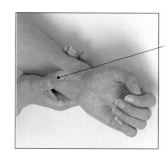

Maintain firm pressure and use a circular motion.

TO RELIEVE MOTION SICKNESS
Place the left thumb on the inside of the right wrist, three finger widths from the center of the wrist crease. Massage between the two tendons for 20 seconds, breathing deeply. Repeat on the other wrist.

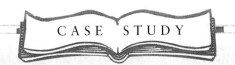
Overcoming Fear of Flying

*Whether it's fear of being in open spaces (agoraphobia) or fear of flying (aerophobia),
a phobia can create an overwhelming sense of panic. To avoid the stress of phobia-triggering
situations, many people curtail their everyday activities. Thanks to stress-reduction techniques
and desensitizing treatment, phobias can be overcome and a normal life resumed.*

Helen is 38 years old and has just been promoted to vice president of sales for her company. Although she is overjoyed, she is suffering a huge amount of stress because she is required to make frequent flights to sales conferences and business meetings. Since her first flight at the age of 19 she has had a tremendous fear of flying. Even before she boards an airplane she sweats profusely, develops palpitations, and feels like she can't breathe—all symptoms of extreme anxiety. On long flights, she tries to calm her nerves by drinking several cocktails, but that makes her feel worse. On her last flight her panic was so great, she realized that unless she faced up to her fear she would have to quit her job.

WHAT SHOULD HELEN DO?

Helen needs to seek help from a qualified therapist who will start her on a course of desensitization. In the process, she will learn how to use deep breathing and relaxation commands in controlled situations designed to trigger her fear. First, Helen will spend time mastering the relaxation commands. Then she will be asked to imagine herself in an airplane and will use the commands to deal with her fright. The next step might be to have her sit in a parked plane. Finally, Helen will use her fear controlling techniques to calm herself during a real flight. While undergoing treatment, it is important that she talk with her boss and explain the problem and how treatment will help.

Action Plan

HEALTH
Learn how to relax and deal with anxiety. Practice deep-breathing techniques. Take a stress management course.

WORK
Inform boss of action being taken for problem. Ask if another manager can go to overseas meetings for the next two months.

LIFESTYLE
Drink calming, caffeine-free herbal teas instead of coffee. Cut down on alcohol consumption, especially on planes. Exercise regularly to relieve stress.

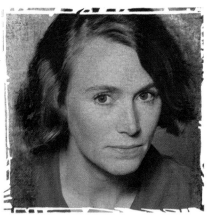

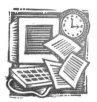

WORK
A fear of flying can jeopardize your job, or even your career, if it is not resolved.

HEALTH
Any kind of extreme fear or phobia can wreak havoc with your physical and mental health.

LIFESTYLE
Anxiety is made worse by stimulants such as caffeine and nicotine. Using alcohol to cope can lead to substance abuse.

HOW THINGS TURNED OUT FOR HELEN

Helen began desensitizing treatment for her phobia. In a few weeks she was able to sit in a flight simulator without suffering any crippling bouts of panic. She also joined a phobia therapy group, which helped her feel less alone with her problem. Helen's first flight went well, but she knows that she will have to practice her relaxation techniques regularly if she wants to hold onto her job and keep her fear of flying in check.

TRAVELING WITHOUT YOUR CHILD

When you go on a trip and leave a small child behind, you can ease anxiety by:

▶ *Discussing the trip with your child, and letting him or her help you prepare a travel plan, perhaps by cutting out pictures of your destination from magazines or brochures.*

▶ *Arranging to have the babysitter take your child to a few special places while you are away.*

▶ *Putting together a package of surprises, one for each day that you will be gone. Include such things as special notes and jokes and small gifts.*

▶ *Making a tape recording of yourself reading one of your child's favorite stories.*

▶ *Marking a calendar with the days you will be away, and asking your youngster to check off each day as it passes.*

TRAVELING WITH CHILDREN

Taking a trip with an infant or young child requires careful planning so that neither of you becomes frazzled along the way. As you make arrangements, try to limit the number of activities and build in some flexibility, allowing extra time to rest, for example, or linger at a favorite spot.

When booking a flight, ask for bulkhead seats. If these are unavailable, request aisle seats to avoid crawling over passengers when your child is restless. If you can travel during off-peak times, your chances are far greater of finding an empty seat for an infant or extra seat space for a toddler to play in.

Before leaving for the airport, always call to find out if the flight is on time. You will save the anguish of coping with a restless youngster if there is a delay.

Whenever possible, plan travel time to coincide with your child's normal sleeping hours; this will limit the amount of time you have to keep him or her occupied.

For waking hours on the road, tie toys for an infant or toddler to the car seat. Provide young children with toys (if possible, include a couple of new ones; these are likely to hold their interest for a longer period than familiar toys), games, and tapes of favorite stories or music.

Those who know how to read can be entertained with games revolving around license plates, such as counting the number of plates from different states that they spot.

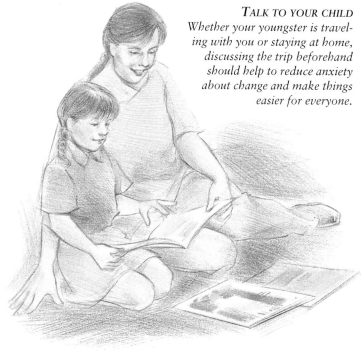

TALK TO YOUR CHILD
Whether your youngster is traveling with you or staying at home, discussing the trip beforehand should help to reduce anxiety about change and make things easier for everyone.

They can also mark on a map the progress to your destination. Plan to stop at least every two hours during a long auto trip, and select a place where children can walk around or run off excess energy.

Children, especially up to the age of six, tend to be more prone to motion sickness than adults. Ask your pediatrician about preventive medication. In a car, it sometimes helps to let the child sit in the front seat, as it is less bumpy than the back.

Feeding wisely

Always carry a varied supply of nutritious snacks and beverages in order to stave off hunger and thirst (and children's attendant crankiness) in case mealtimes are delayed or boredom sets in. Snack foods come in handy even at a restaurant, if you have to wait long for the meal to arrive.

Ask to have your toddler served first, on an airplane or in a restaurant, so you can cut up the food or assist with eating before your own meal arrives. Never permit a child to roam unattended through a restaurant; not only is it extremely annoying to other diners, it could be dangerous if the child accidentally trips a waiter carrying food. It may be necessary for you and your partner to take turns eating while the other takes the young one(s) outside for a stroll.

When traveling by air with an infant, offer a bottle or pacifier during takeoff and landing. Swallowing helps to keep pain-causing pressure from building up in the ears. Having children suck on hard candy or chew gum serves the same purpose.

Sleeping away from home

For the sake of everyone's comfort, stay at hotels or motels that cater to families by providing cribs and possibly babysitting services. As soon as you arrive, put all hazardous or breakable objects out of reach.

Any child may have difficulty sleeping in strange surroundings. It will help if you remember to bring a toy or blanket that the child usually sleeps with and some favorite bedtime storybooks. If you have crossed into a new time zone, expect problems with sleeping routines for at least a day or two.

As difficult as traveling with children can sometimes be, it gives them a chance to explore and adjust to the wider world and helps them develop coping mechanisms that will be valuable to them in the future.

INDEX

—A—

Acupressure
    for anxiety and fatigue 140
    for headaches 23
    for motion sickness 154
Acupuncture 22
Adolescence
    and parents 94
    problems in 60
    see also Family, Parenthood
Adrenaline (epinephrine) 16, 18, 20
    and anger 72
    and immune system 47
    and noise 143
    and sleep 28
Adulthood
    midlife 62
    problems in 61
    A Woman of a Certain
        Age 66
    see also Family, Relationships
Air pollution 144
Alcohol 20
    coping with alcoholism 20
    nonalcoholic drinks 116
    and sleep 28
Alexander Technique 32
Allergies 48
Anger 72
    and driving 150
Anxiety and stress 47, 54
    acupressure for 140
    in children 100
    and earthquakes 144
    and fertility 48, 90
    and job interviews 123
    and noise 143
    and panic attacks 54
    and public speaking 134
    and sex 48, 54
    treatment for 58
Aromatherapy 68
    for alertness 119
    for depression 58
    at home 110
    in sensuous massage 88
    for travel stress 153
Art therapy
    for depression 55
Assertiveness 72
    and anxiety 58
    benefits of 76
    and positive thoughts 44
    questionnaire 76
    and self-defense 146
    techniques 73
    Using Assertion 74
Asthma 48
    and air pollution 144

—B—

Baby
    massage 91
    postpartum depression 91
    see also Pregnancy
Bach flower remedies
    for travel stress 153
Back pain
    chiropractic for 52
    exercise for 31
    fashion and 29
    see also Posture
Bath
    natural 108
    whirlpool 108
Behavior 20
    assertive 73
    of children 100
Bereavement
    A Death in the Family 82
Biochemistry, of stress 17
Biofeedback 38
Biorhythms 143
Blood pressure 16
    see also Hypertension
Blood vessels 18
Body
    flexibility of 34
    posture 29
    relaxation for 39
    types 70
Body language 124
    and assertiveness 73
    do and don't 125
    personal space 125
    and posture 124
    and public speaking 134
    reading the boss 125
Brain 16, 17
    waves 40, 43
Breathing 16
    deep 39
    exercises 135
    rate and noise 143

—C—

Caffeine 27
    and jet lag 152
    and sleep 28
Celebrations
    children's parties 115
    family 114
    party planning 115
    stress-free entertaining 115
    wedding anniversary 116
Child care 94, 136, 137
Children
    and bullying 102

and child care 94
    and danger 145
    illness 102
    motion sickness 156
    parties for 115
    problems of 60, 101
    safe home for 112
    safety measures for 145
    and stress 100
    stresses on 93
    traveling with 156
    traveling without 156
Chiropractic 52
Cholesterol 16, 27
Circulatory problems 47
Communication
    and body language 124
    in the family 79
    for parents 84
    and public speaking 134
    and relationships 84
    at work 122, 132
Commuting 150
Computers
    and eye strain 131
    and lighting 130
    and posture 130
    working with 130
Coping strategies 19, 65
Counseling 58
    Family Therapy 98
    and post-traumatic stress
        disorder 148
    and psychotherapy 145
Crime
    becoming streetwise 146
    and children 145
    prevention 112
    statistics 145
    and traveling 153
    victims of 146
Crying 18

—D—

Danger and stress 16, 17
    in the job 120
Death
    A Death in the Family 82
Deep breathing 39
Depression 55
    aromatherapy for 58
    art therapy for 55
    causes of 55
    after childbirth 91
    coping with 58
    counseling for 58
    and disasters 145
    and light therapy 143
    and negative ions 143

pets for 110
    Seasonal Affective Disorder
        (SAD) 143
    treatment for 58
Diary, stress 20
Diet
    food pyramid 26
    see also Foods
Digestive disorders 48
Disasters 144, 145
    managing trauma 148
Diseases
    caused by stress 47
    Working Up to An Illness 49
    work-related 137
Divorce 81
    dating 81
    A Family Divorce 96
    rates of 78
    remarriage 81
Driving 150
    road rage 150

—E—

Earthquakes 144
Eating, comfort 20, 27
    habits 26
Effects of stress
    on body 16
Emotions 47
    neurotransmitters and 46
Endorphins 18
Energy levels 16, 26
Environment
    at home 104
    noise in 143
    pollution (air and water) 144
    weather 143
    at work 126
    see also Work environment
Events
    stress-causing 16
Exercise
    aerobic 35
    for back pain 31
    benefits of 30
    breathing 135
    for long-distance travel 151
    muscle relaxation 39
    and pulse rate 18
    to relieve anxiety 58
    routines 34, 35
    and sleep 27
    tai chi chuan 36
    see also Fitness
Eye strain
    exercises to relieve 131
    and working with
        computers 131

157

F

Family 78
  celebrations 114
  changes in 78
  dealing with childen 81
  A Death in the Family 82
  extended 78
  A Family Divorce 96
  Family Therapy 98
  medical tree 80
  problems in 79
  time management for 95
  working mother 94
  see also Childhood,
    Adolescence, Adulthood,
    Relationships, Parenthood,
    Divorce
Fats
  and stress 27
  and hypertension 47
Fear of flying 152
  Overcoming a Fear
    of Flying 155
  see also Anxiety
Feng shui
  in the home 106
  in the office 127
Fertility
  and anxiety 48, 90
Fight-or-flight response 16, 18
  and exercise 34
Fitness
  assessing 34
  and pulse rate 18
  see also Exercise
Flexibility 34
Floatation tank 40
Foods
  of love 87
  pyramid 26
  stress-busting 27
  stress-inducing 26
Foot
  massage 28
  reflexology 84
  soak 69
Freud, Sigmund 70

H

Headaches
  acupressure for 23
  homeopathy for 50
Hearing
  stresses on 142
Heart
  attacks and Type A and
    Type B personality 71, 72
  attacks and stress 18
  disease, incidence of 47
  and exercise 30, 34
  problems and stress 47
  rate and driving 150
  rate and noise 143
  rate and stress 16, 18

Herbal remedies
  for motion sickness 154
  for travel stress 153
Home
  air quality in 104
  childproofing 112
  color in 104, 105
  crime prevention 112
  feng shui and 106
  hazards 111
  health spa 108
  lighting in 104
  plants and pets 110
  repairs 110
  safety 111
  scented spray for 110
  smell in 104
  smokers in your 115
  sound 104
Homeopathy 50
  after childbirth 91
  for motion sickness 154
  and public speaking 135
  for travel stress 153
Hormones, stress 16, 17, 18
  and anger 72
  and driving 150
  endorphins 46
  and noise 143
  and sex drive 54
Hostility, *see* Anger
Human Function Curve 47
Hypertension
  and driving 150
  and noise 143
  pets for 110
  and stress 47
Hypnotherapy 43
Hypothalamus 17

I

Illness
  and children 102
  motion sickness 154
  see also Diseases
Immune system
  anxiety and fear 47
  and stress 18, 27, 46, 47, 48
Infertility 48, 90
Injuries
  work-related 137
Insomnia 27, 28
  hops pillow 28
  lavender pillow 101
  remedies for 28

J

Jet lag 152
Jobs
  changing 122
  choosing 122
  combating job stress 119, 120
  and depression 55
  dressing for 123

elements of stress in 119, 132
  interviews 123
  loss of 140
  maternity leave 136
  An Out-of-Work
    Executive 138
  personality and 118
  Potential Stress Factor of 120
  reading the boss 125
  self-employed 128
  suitable 122
  see also Work
Jung, Carl 70

L

Laughter
  and stress 18
Life events 19, 64
  Social Readjustment
    Rating Scale 19

M

Marriage
  and attraction 84
  bliss 86
  staying together 85
  see also Divorce, Family
Massage 28
  baby 91
  face 109
  foot 28
  legs 109
  reflexology 84
  sensuous 88
  at work 119
Meditation 42
  tai chi chuan 36
Menstruation 48
Middle age
  problems in 62
  A Woman of a Certain Age 66
Mind
  and depression 55
  overcoming stress 48
  and visualization 135, 147
Monitoring stress 20
  Monthly Stress Test 24
Motion sickness 154
Muscle tension 16, 29
  and back pain 31
  chiropractic for 52
  foot massage for 28
  and long distance travel 151
  and massage 119
  relaxation for 39
  shoulder stretch 53, 129
  and visualization 147

N

Natural therapies 48
  acupuncture 22
  Alexander Technique 32
  for anxiety and depression 58

aromatherapy 68
  art therapy 55
  biofeedback 38
  chiropractic 52
  effects on stress 48
  feng shui 106, 127
  holistic approach 48
  homeopathy 50
  reflexology 84
  tai chi chuan 36
  visualization 147
  yin and yang balls 140
  yoga 56
Nervous system 17
  and noise 143
Noise pollution 142
Noradrenaline (norepinephrine) 16
  and immune system 47
  and noise 143
Nutrition 26
  effects of stress on 27

O

Old age
  deterioration in 80
  and family 79
  problems in 63
  safe home for 111

P

Panic attacks 54
  and public speaking 135
  see also Anxiety
Parenthood 90
  and communication 94
  maternity leave 136
  The Perfect Mother 21
  quality time 93
  A Single Parent 92
  spending time with children 93
  stresses on children 93
  and teenagers 94
  work and 94, 95, 136
  see also Childhood,
    Adolescence, Family
Parties
  planning 115
Performance
  and stress 18, 47
Personality 19
  and health 71
  and job choice 122
  and personal space 125
  and relationships 84
  types 70, 71
Personal Space 125
Personal Stressful Event Scale 64
Pets
  in the home 110
  therapy 104
Phobia
  Overcoming a Fear of
    Flying 155
Physical responses to stress 16, 17

Physical signs of stress 19
Pineal gland 143
Pituitary gland 17
Plants 110
  and feng shui 106, 127
  at home 106
  in the office 126
Pollution
  air 143
  noise 143
  water 144
Positive thinking 44, 149
  for drivers 150
Posture 29, 30
  Alexander Technique 32
  and body language 124
  correction of 48
  lifting and carrying 30
  and repetitive stress
    injury (RSI) 30
  and self-confidence 29
  and sitting 30
  and working with computers
    130
Pregnancy and stress 72, 90
  homeopathy after childbirth 91
  maternity leave 126
  postpartum depression 91
Public speaking 134
  and breathing exercises 135
  golden rules of 134
  and visualization 135
Public transportation
  see Commuting
Pulse rate 34

——— R ———

Reflexology 84
  for couples 84
Relationships 84
  communication in 84
  coping with pressures 86
  disagreements in 86
  factors that affect 85
  foods of love 87
  reflexology for 84
  sensuous massage 88
  at work 136
  see also Family
Relaxation
  bath for 108
  changes in body with 38
  deep 40, 41
  floatation tank 40
  massage for 119
  meditation 42
  methods of 38
  muscle 39
  music for 41
  response 40
  retreats 48
  sensory deprivation for 40
  and television 38
  unwinding from work 104
  visualization for 147

Repetitive stress injury (RSI) 30
  and computers 131
Reproductive problems 48
  infertility 90
Responses to stress
  emotional 47
  inappropriate 20
  physical 16, 17
  trauma 148
Retirement 137
  forced 140
  problems in 63
  see also Jobs, Work
Retreats 48
Risks, taking 20
Road rage 150

——— S ———

Safety
  for children 145
  while driving 151
  at home 111
  streetwise 146
Seasonal Affective Disorder
  (SAD) 143
Selye, Hans 17, 19
Serotonin
  and depression 46, 55
Sex drive
  and anxiety 48
  and stress 54
  see also Relationships
Skin disorders 48
Sleep
  and alcohol 28
  away from home 156
  beds 27
  and caffeine 28
  for children 101
  deprivation and stress 27
  and exercise 27
  foot massage for 28
  insomnia 27, 28, 101
  and jet lag 152
  and long-distance travel 151
  and smoking 28
Smoking
  passive 115
  to relieve stress 20
  and sleep 28
Social Readjustment Rating
  Scale 19
Stress
  -busting foods 27
  causes of 19
  and chemical and nervous
    system responses 17
  effects on body 16
  effects on performance 18
  inappropriate responses to 20
  -inducing foods 26
  and life problems 60
  monitoring 20
  Personal Stressful Event
    Scale 64

Social Readjustment Rating
  Scale 19
  symptoms and signs of 19
  testing 24, 64
  treatment of -related illness 48
Stroke and stress 18
Sugar, blood 26
Symptoms
  of depression 55
  Monthly Stress Test 24
  of post-traumatic stress
    disorder (PTSD) 148
  of stress 19

——— T ———

Tai chi chuan 36
Thrill seeking 20
Time management 133
  for family 95
  organization 133
  planning ahead 132
  for self-employed 128
Traffic jam 150
Trauma
  post-traumatic stress disorder
    (PTSD) 48
  Post-Traumatic Stress Victim 149
  treating 148
  see also Disasters
Travel
  abroad 153
  air 152
  car safety 151
  with children 156
  without children 156
  exercises for 151
  fear of flying 152
  long distance 151
  motion sickness 154
  natural therapies for travel
    stress 153
  on public transportation 150
  vacation checklist 153
  see also Commuting

——— U ———

Ulcers
  and Helicobacter pylori 48
  and stress 48

——— V ———

Vacation 152
Violence
  domestic 145
  street 146
Visualization 147
  in sport competitions 40, 41
  exercise 147
  for job interviews 123
  for public speaking 135
  for relaxation 40
  for stressful situations 124
  technique 41, 147

——— W ———

Water
  pollution 144
  purification 144
Weather
  and depression 143
  Seasonal Affective Disorder
    (SAD) 143
White noise
  and insomnia 28
  and noise pollution 143
Women
  maternity leave 136
  The Perfect Mother 21
  see also Family, Pregnancy
Work
  assertion at 74
  and business plans 129
  and child care 136, 137
  causes of stress at 118
  communication at 131
  and computers 130
  dealing with people at 133
  delegating 132
  and eye strain 131
  getting home after 104
  and health problems 118
  at home 128
  ideal workstation 130
  and lighting 130
  massage at 119
  maternity leave 136
  networking 128
  and planning ahead 132
  posture at 30
  reducing stress at 119
  and repetitive stress
    injury (RSI) 131
  retirement 137
  stress-beaters at 131
  stress-free home office 129
  stress-related diseases and
    illnesses 137
  stretches at 129
  see also Computers, Jobs,
    Time management, Work
    environment
Work environment
  feng shui and 127
  ionizers for 127
  physical stressors in 126
  power of plants 126
  sick building syndrome 126
  ventilation 127

——— Y ———

Yin and yang balls 140
Yoga
  to reduce stress 56

Acknowledgements

Carroll & Brown Limited
would like to thank
Ellen Dupont
Sue Mims
Irena Hoare

John Wiley & Sons, New York
Mosby, St. Louis

Penguin Books, London (chart, pages 64–65)
International Management & Reed Business Publishing (chart, page 118)

Additional design assistance
Richard Horsford
Paola Bernardi

Additional editorial assistance
Ian Wood

Advice and assistance
Ainsworths Homoeopathic Pharmacy
Aquatonics
Bundeskriminalamtes
Bureau of Justice Statistics
Central Statistical Office
Department of the Environment
Feng Shui Society
Institute of Environmental Health Officers
Institut National de la Statistique et des Etudes Economiques
Keep Able
National Center for Health Statistics
National Highway Traffic Safety Administration
National Institute for Occupational Safety and Health
Statistical Office of the European Committee
Statistisches Bundesamt
SW2000 Teleworking Studies
Tim Harper, The College of Osteopaths
Wingfield Chiropractic Clinic

Photograph sources
8 Range/Bettmann
10 Popperfoto
11 Gregg deGuire/London Features
13 (Top) Popperfoto; (Bottom) Robin Kaplan/London Features
14 Range/Bettmann
17 Tony Stone Images
18 Sally and Richard Greenhill
20 Tony Stone Images
22 Wellcome Institute Library, London
32 S.T.A.T.
34 Peter Tizzard
36 (Bottom) Eye Ubiquitous
38 Zefa
40 (Top) Tony Stone Images; (Bottom) Courtesy Float Systems Int. (London)/Tony Isbitt
41 James Watt/Planet Earth Pictures
42 Robert Harding Picture Library
43 Sarah Errington/Hutchison Library
50 Peter Tizzard
52 Scofield Chiropractic Clinic
55 (Left) Peter Tizzard; (Right) 'Art as Healing,' Edward Adamson
56 Reed International Books Ltd./Hawkley Studios
71 Mary Evans Picture Library
78 Mary Evans Picture Library
90 Petit Format/Nestlé/SPL
99 Zefa
100 John Walmsley
102 (Left) Bubbles/Pauline Cutler; (Right) Mary Evans Picture Library
106 The Feng Shui Network/Harry Archer
108 Thalgo UK Ltd.
114 Zefa
127 Drawing after a building by R. H. Partnership Architects with Battle McCarthy
134 Range/Bettmann

142 Robert Harding Picture Library/Earl J. Young
143 Full Spectrum Lighting Ltd.
144 Robert Harding Picture Library/Explorer
150 (Top) Eye Ubiquitous; (Bottom) Autosport Photographic

Illustrators
Joanna Cameron
Jane Craddock-Watson
Eugene Fleury
John Geary
Christine Pilsworth
Paul Williams
Angela Wood

Charts
Clive Bruton
Lee Maunder
Nick Roland

Photographic assistance
Nick Allen
Ian Boddy
Alex Hansen
Sid Sideris

Make-up
Bettina Graham
Juliana Mendes Ebden

Picture researcher
Sandra Schneider

Research
Laura Price

Index
Sharon Freed